Contents

About the authors

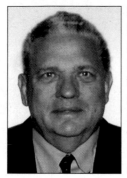

Stephen R. Kaplan is Professor Emeritus of Clinical Medicine at the Brown University Medical School in Providence, Rhode Island. Having trained in Clinical Pharmacology and Therapeutics, Dr. Kaplan was Professor of Medicine at Brown where he initiated and led the Division of Rheumatology for two decades. Subsequently, he became Professor of Medicine at the State University of New York at Buffalo where he led the development of the Division of General Internal Medicine. He has also served as a Scholar-in- Residence at the Kettering Foundation in Health Policy.

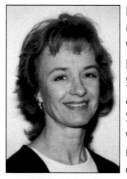

Doctor Jennifer G. Worrall is Consultant Rheumatologist at the Whittington Hospital NHS Trust, London, England and Honorary Senior Lecturer at the Royal Free and University College Medical School, London, England. Her work covers all aspects of general rheumatology. Other interests are clinical effectiveness and scientific methodology.

Introduction

The musculoskeletal system

The musculoskeletal system, which enables us to move around consists of the bones, joints, and muscles of the body. All sorts of problems may develop in this system, particularly as we get older. Although only three percent of people under 60 years old have joint pain or stiffness, the figure rises to almost 50 percent in people aged over 75.

What is arthritis and rheumatism?

"Arthritis" refers to problems with the joints. There are many forms of arthritis, ranging from mild to serious, and not all of them get progressively worse. "Rheumatism" is a vaguer term with no precise medical meaning, which refers generally to aches and pains, and problems with the soft tissues, such as muscles and tendons, rather than with the joints.

The aim of this book is to help you understand how your musculoskeletal system works, what can go wrong with it, and what help is available if it does. We hope, especially, to show you that there is a lot you can

The human skeleton

The human skeleton is able to move so well because it has many joints. These tend to degenerate over time and can cause pain and discomfort.

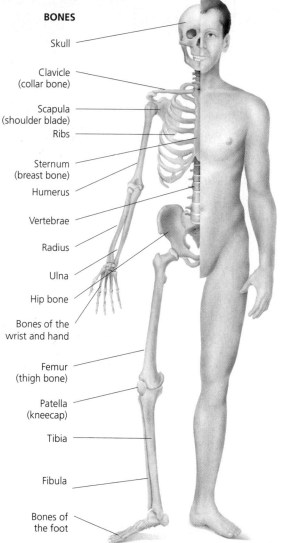

BONES

Skull

Clavicle
(collar bone)

Scapula
(shoulder blade)

Ribs

Sternum
(breast bone)

Humerus

Vertebrae

Radius

Ulna

Hip bone

Bones of the
wrist and hand

Femur
(thigh bone)

Patella
(kneecap)

Tibia

Fibula

Bones of
the foot

do to help yourself, both to treat problems when they arise and to prevent them occurring.

The problems of arthritis and rheumatism are not confined to older people—many common conditions affect people of all ages. Even people who do not have problems can learn to look after their joints better and so avoid problems in the future. So we hope you will find something of interest to you, whatever your age and whether or not you have arthritis. On page 112, you will find a list of addresses for further information.

How your joints work
Synovial joints

Joints hold the bones together and generally allow movement. Some joints, such as those in the pelvis, do not move very much and those in your skull do not move at all. But many joints can move freely and those that do are called "synovial joints." All of the most important joints in the body are of this type and have the same basic structure (see below). They are capable of a wide range of movement and come in many different shapes and sizes—compare the joints in your finger with those in your knees, for example; the joints look different but consist of the same basic elements.

The ends of the two bones forming the joint are covered by cartilage. This is a sort of gristle that acts as a shock absorber and helps the bones to move smoothly over each other. The bones are held together by very strong ligaments and the whole joint is contained in a bag called a "capsule." The inside of the capsule is covered with a lining called "synovium' (hence the name "synovial joint") which forms a slippery surface and so allows the joint to move easily. The joint capsule contains a small amount of lubricating

Synovial joints

Although the synovial joints in your body come in a wide range of shapes and sizes, they are nevertheless made up of the same basic elements.

Bone – hard framework that supports and protects tissues

Synovium – secretes the synovial fluid

Synovial fluid – lubricates the joint capsule

Ligaments – hold the bones together and form the capsule

Cartilage – protects the ends of the bones

liquid, called "synovial fluid," that is produced by the synovium.

When a joint moves, the muscles and tendons around it need to slide easily over each other and this smooth action is helped by structures called "bursas." A bursa is a flattened sac, rather like a balloon before it has been inflated. It contains a small amount of synovial fluid, which makes the internal surfaces slippery and allows them to slide over each other. Many tendons run in lubricated sheaths, also lined by synovium (see diagram on page 6).

Smooth joint movement: bursas and synovial fluid

Left knee, seen from the left side. Bursas are flattened sacs, containing synovial fluid which makes them slippery, allowing the muscles and tendons to slide easily over each other when the joint moves.

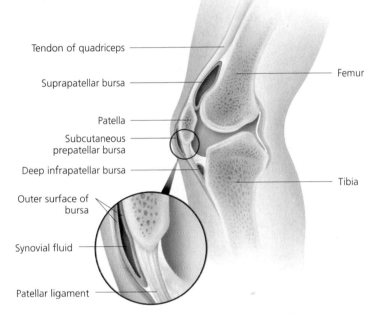

Tendon of quadriceps

Suprapatellar bursa

Patella

Subcutaneous prepatellar bursa

Deep infrapatellar bursa

Outer surface of bursa

Synovial fluid

Patellar ligament

Femur

Tibia

Case history: Alan

Alan went to his internist because he started feeling a pain in his groin whenever he walked any distance, and thought he might have developed a hernia. After examining him, Alan's doctor found that his right hip was rather stiff and sent him for an X-ray. This showed that, at 70, Alan had mild osteoarthritis in his right hip joint. His primary care physician advised him to take simple painkillers when necessary but stressed the

Tendons

Many tendons run in lubricated sheaths, also lined by synovium, and lubricated by synovial fluid. The sheaths of the underside of the right hand are shown in blue.

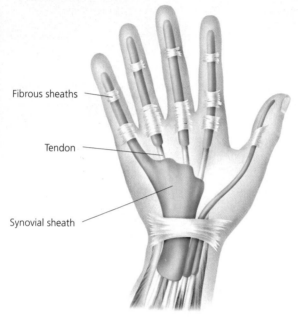

Fibrous sheaths

Tendon

Synovial sheath

importance of keeping active and taking regular exercise. Alan joined an over-50s swimming group at a fitness club and, after a few weeks of regular sessions, he found the groin pain much less troublesome.

Case history: Cathy

Cathy was just 35 when she noticed that her hands were becoming swollen and painful. She also felt tired and listless and very stiff all over her body first thing in the morning. After about six weeks, it was taking her an hour and a half to be up and about in the morning, and this was a problem since she needed to get her children off to school. She saw her internist and eventually investigations revealed that she had rheumatoid arthritis. Cathy was referred to a rheumatologist, a specialist in diseases of the joints, who started her on drugs to ease the pain and swelling and slow the progress of her condition. Cathy was also asked to visit with a physiotherapist, who advised her on suitable exercise to keep her joints working, and she saw an occupational therapist, who advised her on ways of performing daily tasks that would reduce the strain on her joints. She was also scheduled to see a physician regularly for monitoring and, after a few weeks, her symptoms were far less of a problem than before.

KEY POINTS

- Arthritis is very common and there are many different types

- A lot of help—including self-help—is available for arthritis sufferers

- All joints that move freely have the same basic structure

- The soft tissues of which a joint consists— ligaments, cartilage, capsule, and the lining of the joint or synovium—are just as important as the bones

Getting a diagnosis

What are the symptoms?

When your musculoskeletal system goes wrong, you feel pain and stiffness and you may notice swelling of your joints. Symptoms can be very troublesome, even disabling, and can sometimes be out of all proportion to the seriousness of the condition.

Pain, in particular, is a complex symptom and can be made much worse by stress, anxiety, or depression. It is important to recognize these influences and not just assume that your arthritis must be getting worse.

Expectations can also play a part here. If you watched an older relative gradually become disabled by painful arthritis, perhaps in the days before there were effective treatments, then, at the first sign of the inevitable aches and pains of middle age, you might become worried that the same fate awaits you. Your anxiety and distress would make your pain much worse, and pain is by far the most disabling symptom—joints that are structurally sound may be almost useless if every movement causes severe pain. Fortunately, we now understand a great deal about joint symptoms and arthritis, and we have lots of treatments and advice to help sufferers lead normal lives.

When you visit your doctor with pain, stiffness, or swelling of a joint, your doctor will need quite a lot of information from you and may order various tests to establish the cause of the problem. Pain in or around a joint (known medically as "arthralgia") doesn't necessarily mean that you have arthritis. Other diseases can produce this kind of symptom. Flu, for example, can cause severe aches in the joints and muscles but the pain disappears as you recover.

Seeing the doctor
Taking your history

When you first talk to a doctor about your problems, he or she will check your symptoms and your past record of health. This is called "taking your history."

Your doctor will also want to know whether any close relatives have arthritis. Your family history is relevant because some people inherit a genetic susceptibility to some forms of arthritis. You should also tell your doctor if you have had any past injury to the joint, because this may cause problems to develop later, in and around joints.

Certain other conditions may be associated with the onset of arthritis, such as the skin disease psoriasis or the bowel condition ulcerative colitis. Sometimes, arthritis can follow an infection. This is referred to as "reactive arthritis." It is important to mention any recent foreign travel in case you may have picked up an infection that could account for your symptoms.

Try to be as specific as you can when describing your symptoms—when they began, whether anything triggered them, whether they are constant or intermittent, whether anything makes them better or worse, what treatment you have tried so far, and what effect it had, including side effects.

Physical examination

Your doctor may need to examine you thoroughly, even if you have only a single painful joint, because other joints may be similarly affected, even if they are not painful at the moment. Sometimes, a problem in one joint can cause strain in nearby joints.

Although these joints are normal, they become painful. For example, shoulder pain may be caused by a problem in the neck, back pain can arise from knee or hip problems, which are affecting the way you walk, and your knee may hurt even though the real problem is actually in your hip joint.

During the examination, your doctor will be looking for swelling, tenderness, stiffness of the joint, and whether the joint is stable. This involves checking the muscles and ligaments that hold the joint in position. Your doctor may also take the opportunity to make other routine checks, such as measuring your blood pressure.

Tests and investigations

Very often, your doctor will be able to identify your problem without the need for any tests, especially if only one joint is painful or if the diagnosis is obvious and straightforward. Otherwise, the tests you have will depend on individual circumstances, but may include some or all of the following.

Blood tests

Full blood count

A machine counts the number of red and white blood cells and platelets in a cubic millimeter of blood. The

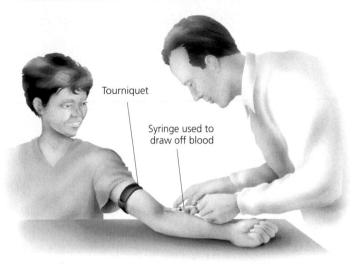

Tourniquet

Syringe used to
draw off blood

A blood test can provide your doctor with a great deal of
information to assist with diagnosis.

hemoglobin level in the red blood cells is also
measured. This shows whether you are anemic, as can
happen in rheumatoid arthritis. Anemia is a disorder in
which hemoglobin (the oxygen-carrying component of
red blood cells) is deficient or abnormal. A full blood
count also measures the number of white cells in the
blood, which often increase when there is an infection.

Erythrocyte sedimentation rate (ESR)

Blood consists of cells and fluid (plasma). The most
numerous blood cells are the red blood cells that
transport oxygen around the body. The ESR measures
the "stickiness" of the red blood cells. A raised ESR
suggests that inflammation is present, although it gives
no indication as to the cause. The ESR is raised in those
types of arthritis where the joints are severely inflamed.
In osteoarthritis, the commonest form of arthritis,

inflammation is absent or mild and the ESR tends to be normal.

Uric acid
This is the substance that forms crystals in the joints during attacks of gout. The level of uric acid in the blood is often raised in people who suffer with gout.

Rheumatoid factor
Rheumatoid factor is an antibody that appears in the blood in some people with rheumatoid arthritis. It can also be found in low levels in normal people, especially as they get older, and in some relatives of people with rheumatoid arthritis. Rheumatoid factor does not cause disease but it can be a useful marker.

X-rays
X-rays are not always needed to make a diagnosis of arthritis. Most people over the age of 50 have some degree of osteoarthritis and joint pain is not always related to changes seen on the X-ray.

Most forms of arthritis begin by affecting the soft tissues of the joint, such as the cartilage in osteoarthritis and the synovium in rheumatoid arthritis. Soft tissues are not easily seen on an X-ray. The X-ray is of most use in showing whether the arthritis has progressed to affect the bones and as a baseline against which future changes can be measured.

The X-ray of a joint affected by arthritis may show the following changes:

Reduced joint space
The space between the bones of the joint is normally filled with cartilage, which cannot be seen on an X-ray.

X-ray investigation

An X-ray is of the most use in showing whether the arthritis has progressed to affect the bones; it also provides a baseline against which future changes can be measured.

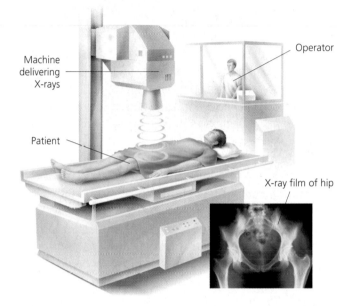

Machine delivering X-rays

Operator

Patient

X-ray film of hip

In many forms of arthritis, the cartilage becomes thinner and the joint space narrows.

Erosions

These are holes in the bones of the joint and they occur in advanced arthritis. Erosions can occur in rheumatoid arthritis and other forms of arthritis where the joints are severely inflamed.

Bony overgrowth (osteophytes)

Sometimes, arthritis causes extra bone to grow at the edges of affected joints. This can be seen quite clearly on an X-ray. In the spine, the extra bone can cause pinching of a nerve, leading to pain along the route of the nerve.

Putting it all together

A careful history and examination, together with a few simple tests, are often all your internist needs in order to make a diagnosis. Sometimes this is not possible and you will need to see a specialist in joint and bone disorders. However, even the specialist may not be able to make a diagnosis on the first consultation and the full picture becomes clear only with the passage of time. You will be given treatment to ease your pain and stiffness. A period of observation, perhaps with a repeat of some of the tests, can help to establish a diagnosis.

The specialist you see may be a rheumatologist who specializes in inflammatory disease and the medical treatment of arthritis and rheumatism. Or he or she may be an orthopedic surgeon if your problems are the result of injury or mechanical damage rather than inflammatory disease.

KEY POINTS

- A careful history and examination help your doctor to make a diagnosis

- Blood tests and X-rays may help but they are not always needed

Osteoarthritis

How common is osteoarthritis?

Osteoarthritis is very common and affects most of us as we get older. It is the most common form of arthritis in people over the age of 65. Men are more likely to be affected than women before they reach 45, but, in the over-55s, the balance shifts so that more women are affected.

Osteoarthritis is sometimes called "wear-and-tear arthritis" and "degenerative arthritis," but wear and-tear and degeneration are not the whole story. Lots of people who have done heavy work all their lives do not develop osteoarthritis and it is not restricted to older people.

Does it run in families?

Osteoarthritis can run in families and, if your parents had it, you have a slightly greater chance of developing it too. It can also develop early in any joint that has previously been seriously injured. Football, soccer, and hockey players, for instance, often suffer repeated cartilage injuries and may develop osteoarthritis in their knees. Besides the knee, osteoarthritis is common in the hip, the joint at the base of the thumb or big toe, the spine, especially the lower back, and the neck.

What's happening?

Osteoarthritis was once seen as a natural and inevitable consequence of aging, but we now know that the real picture is rather more complex. Doctors now think that osteoarthritis may be a disorder affecting the cells responsible for making cartilage. The cartilage loses its slippery surface, cracks develop, and it becomes roughened (see diagram opposite).

Over time, the cartilage becomes thinner and the joint may not move as freely as it once did. The bone at the edges of the joint may change shape and bony lumps, or osteophytes, may form. In advanced cases, the cartilage may disappear entirely and the bones forming the joint may become deformed.

Women who have a family history of the condition are likely to develop problems in the joints of their fingers and thumbs, and in their knees. In some people, joint problems are more widespread, with hands, feet, hips, knees, and shoulders all being affected. Sometimes, a single joint, such as the knee, may be the only one affected, especially if it has been previously injured.

Symptoms

Many people have no symptoms at all and find out that they have osteoarthritis only when an X-ray is taken for some other reason. Most people, however, show some symptoms (see page 18).

Despite their gnarled appearance and the stiffness and pain, arthritic joints can continue to have good function and support.

Osteoarthritis – what is going on?

Osteoarthritis is often referred to as wear and tear of the joints.

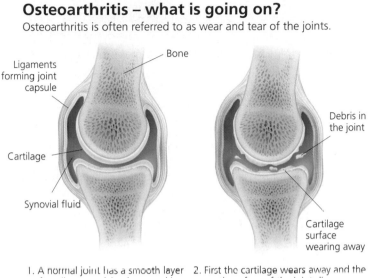

Ligaments forming joint capsule

Bone

Cartilage

Synovial fluid

Debris in the joint

Cartilage surface wearing away

1. A normal joint has a smooth layer of cartilage overlying bone and is lubricated by synovial fluid

2. First the cartilage wears away and the smooth surface of the joint disappears; small pieces of the cartilage may break off, creating debris in the joint which can interrupt movement

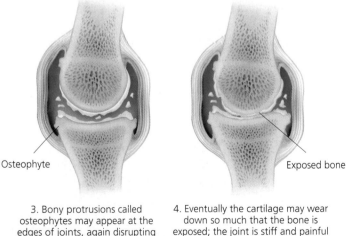

Osteophyte

Exposed bone

3. Bony protrusions called osteophytes may appear at the edges of joints, again disrupting function and causing pain

4. Eventually the cartilage may wear down so much that the bone is exposed; the joint is stiff and painful and may be swollen with excess synovial fluid

Common symptoms in osteoarthritis

- The joint is painful after exercise and at the end of the day, but the pain gets better with rest.
- The joint is stiff first thing in the morning or after a daytime rest, but quickly loosens up with exercise.
- The joint creaks or grinds when you move it—this is known as "crepitus." Crepitus is often not painful and should not prevent you from using the joint.
- Tender lumps may appear on the small joints at the ends of your fingers and the bases of your thumbs.

Occasionally these joints, especially the knees, may suddenly become swollen and very painful, especially after some vigorous activity, such as an unusually long walk. The inflammation is usually mild and should respond to an anti-inflammatory drug and a short period of rest. Sometimes, the excess fluid in the joint needs to be drained and an injection of steroid given to reduce the inflammation.

Arthritis in the neck may cause irritation of a nerve root, leading to numbness, pins-and-needles, and pain in the arms. Headaches can also occur and are the result of tension in the muscles at the back of the neck. Dizziness on looking up may be caused by pressure on some of the blood vessels that supply the brain.

Diagnosis

Usually, your doctor will be able to tell whether you have osteoarthritis after he or she has taken your history and examined you, as described on pages 9–10. Sometimes an X-ray will be needed. Osteoarthritis does not show up as abnormalities in blood tests (see pages 10–12).

Treatment

The mainstays of treatment for osteoarthritis are:

- exercise
- reducing the strain on the affected joints and
- painkillers when necessary.

The right kind of exercise will maintain movement and strengthen the muscles around a joint. This will stabilize the joint and protect it from strain.

If you are overweight, then losing some weight will help to take the strain off your lower back, knees, ankles, and feet.

Painkillers and sometimes anti-inflammatory drugs can relieve the pain and stiffness and allow you to benefit fully from an exercise program.

For more detailed information on exercise, see pages 94–103, and for more information on treatment, turn to page 71.

The outlook

The idea that disability caused by osteoarthritis is inevitable as we get older is old-fashioned. Although getting older is, of course, inevitable, disability is most definitely not inevitable. Modern medicine has a lot to offer and there is also a great deal you can do to help yourself. If you learn to use your joints appropriately, you can remain healthy and active into old age. The way to do this is to avoid straining the joints but you need to take regular exercise, maintain an ideal weight, and use painkillers when necessary.

Sometimes, joints become so damaged, painful, and stiff that they can no longer work properly, in spite of regular exercise and painkillers. The cartilage becomes thin and disappears completely and bone rubs over bone, instead of on cartilage. The joint may be painful all the time, even when it is held still and rested. Surgery to remove the worn-out joint and replace it with an artificial one may have to be the answer.

Artificial hips and knees have been available for over 20 years and many thousands of these operations are performed every year, with a very high success rate. Indeed, joint replacement surgery is probably the greatest advance ever made in the treatment of arthritis!

KEY POINTS

- Osteoarthritis affects most of us as we get older

- You will keep more active by avoiding straining the joints, exercising, keeping your weight down, and using painkillers when the need arises

Rheumatoid arthritis

What is rheumatoid arthritis?

Rheumatoid arthritis is quite different from osteoarthritis. It is caused by an intense inflammation in the synovial joints and it can arise at any time from the teenage years onward. It is more common in women and the peak age of onset is between 30 and 50. Rheumatoid arthritis is the most common form of inflammatory arthritis and it affects one to two percent of the population. Even so, it is much less common than osteoarthritis which affects almost all of us to some degree as we get older.

Rheumatoid arthritis should really be called "rheumatoid disease" because not only the joints but other parts of the body may be affected—for example, the skin, lungs, and eyes. As it is such a complex, widespread disease with many effects, rheumatoid arthritis is usually treated by specialists known as rheumatologists. Rheumatologists may be in private practice, or in specialized hospital centers.

What's happening?

Rheumatoid arthritis is one of a group of conditions called "autoimmune connective tissue diseases." The other conditions in this group are much rarer. In all of these conditions, the body's immune system is overactive and appears to attack the body's own tissues. Something must trigger this process—for example, a virus or a toxin—but at the moment we do not know what it is.

A great deal of research is directed at finding the trigger with the hope of then developing a cure for the condition. But, although we do not have a cure at the present time, we have treatments that are very effective at suppressing the overactivity of the immune system and keeping the process under control.

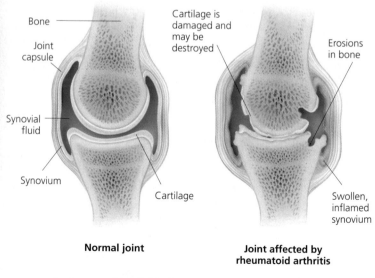

Bone

Joint capsule

Synovial fluid

Synovium

Cartilage is damaged and may be destroyed

Erosions in bone

Cartilage

Swollen, inflamed synovium

Normal joint

Joint affected by rheumatoid arthritis

In rheumatoid arthritis the synovium, which lines the joint capsule, becomes swollen and inflamed. The inflammation can damage the cartilage and bone.

We may not know the cause of rheumatoid arthritis but we understand many of the changes that take place in the tissues as the disease progresses. We know that the seat of the inflammation is the synovium, the slippery lining of joints, tendon sheaths, and bursas. The synovium becomes swollen and thickened and may produce large amounts of synovial fluid. Cartilage and ligaments may be damaged and eventually the bone also may be damaged, forming cavities called "erosions."

In rare cases, the joint may eventually be destroyed. In severe cases, the inflammation may affect other parts of the body, such as the eyes, skin, and lungs.

Symptoms

The symptoms of rheumatoid arthritis are varied and may begin quite suddenly (see box).

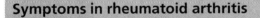

Symptoms in rheumatoid arthritis

- Many joints are affected at the same time with swelling, warmth, and tenderness.
- The hands and feet are the most common joints involved, followed by the wrists, ankles, knees, shoulders, and neck.
- When the inflammation is active, fever, loss of appetite, and weight loss are common.
- Many people feel tired and lacking in energy because they are also anemic.
- Severe stiffness early in the morning which tends to ease as the day progresses but may last for many hours.

In severe cases, morning stiffness seems to affect every joint in the body. Many people say that this stiffness and difficulty in getting moving is more disabling than the pain. The inflammation may affect parts of the body outside the joints. The eye may become red and sore and if this happens you will need to see an ophthalmologist. Your lungs may be affected and you should always report any increase in breathlessness to your doctor. Small blood vessels can become inflamed (a condition known as "vasculitis"), causing rashes and sometimes ulcers.

Rheumatoid nodules

Some people develop nodules under the skin at sites of friction, such as the feet, the backs of the heels, the backs of the hands, and the elbows. The nodules are painless and, apart from being unsightly, do not usually cause trouble. Occasionally, they grow to a large size and interfere with the wearing of shoes. The nodules are easily removed by minor surgery but this is avoided as far as possible, as they tend to recur.

Later symptoms

Very occasionally, the symptoms of rheumatoid arthritis improve on their own after the first few weeks or months, but most people need treatment. Rheumatoid arthritis usually follows a pattern of "remissions," followed by "relapses" or "flares." Remissions are good periods when the symptoms are less troublesome and relapses are when the inflammation is more active.

The aim of treatment is to control the relapses and maintain, or prolong, the remissions. Often, remissions can last for many years.

Who's who in the care of progressive rheumatoid arthritis:

- The rheumatologist, who is in overall charge, selects and monitors the appropriate drugs, and coordinates the input of the other specialists. In a hospital setting, you may also sometimes see other members of the specialist's team, such as a fellow in rheumatology or a resident physician.

- A rheumatology nurse specialist may see you while your condition is in a stable phase to monitor your drug therapy. He or she is also a valuable contact for extra advice and information.

- The physiotherapist plays a vital role in relieving symptoms and preserving muscle strength and movement of affected joints. He or she may recommend splints for affected joints from time-to-time to protect them and maintain their correct position, and will also advise on the right sort of exercises for you to perform at home.

- The occupational therapist is concerned with keeping you functioning as normally as possible and can advise on how to perform everyday activities most efficiently without straining the joints. He or she can also advise on aids and appliances.

- A podiatrist may be needed if you develop foot problems, such as toe deformities, calluses, and ulcers.

- An orthopedic surgeon will become involved if surgery, such as joint replacement, is being considered.

- Social workers can advise on the wide range of help that is available through the social services resources of your particular community.

Diagnosis

A detailed history, a careful examination, and some simple blood tests are usually all that are needed for an experienced doctor to make a diagnosis of rheumatoid arthritis. A complete blood count will show whether you are anemic (a reduced number of red blood cells, common in rheumatoid arthritis) and an erythrocyte sedimentation rate (ESR) will show whether inflammation is present.

A test for rheumatoid factor (see page 12) may help in the diagnosis. X-rays often appear normal in the early stages of the disease but they should be taken so that they can be used as a baseline against which to compare later X-rays. A chest X-ray and X-rays of the hands and feet are the most useful.

Treatment

The aims underlying treatment for rheumatoid arthritis are to:

- relieve symptoms
- preserve muscle strength and joint movement
- protect the joints from further damage
- help the individual to lead as normal a life as possible.

At a specialized center, you will meet with a number of specialists, each of whom can help in a different way (see page 25).

Drug treatments

Several different types of drugs are used to treat rheumatoid arthritis. First and very important are non-steroidal anti-inflammatory drugs (NSAIDs) and analgesics (painkillers). They are dealt with in the section on drugs on page 71 but, briefly, anti-inflammatory drugs reduce pain, stiffness, and swelling, whereas analgesics provide added pain relief if this is necessary. Although these drugs can help the symptoms of rheumatoid arthritis, they do not have any effect on the long-term progression of the disease.

The second and equally important group of drugs that help to prevent joint damage includes methotrexate, sulphasalazine, azathioprine, leflunomide (Arava), gold salts, penicillamine, and hydroxychloroquine.

Each of these medications, known collectively as "disease-modifying anti-rheumatoid drugs" or "DMARDs" (pronounced "deemards") (see box on page 28) has been shown to improve the long-term outcome in people with rheumatoid arthritis. These drugs are chemically very different from each other—we do not yet know in detail how they work but they have some shared features.

Several new DMARDs work directly on the immune system. Examples are etanercept (Enbrel), infliximab (Remicade), and adalimumab (Humira). They are powerful drugs that are given by injection and need to be closely monitored. Long-term effects are not yet clear so they are reserved for people with severe rheumatoid arthritis who have not been helped by other DMARDs.

Steroids can be useful in treating rheumatoid arthritis because they have a powerful anti-inflammatory action. They may be given in pill form or by injection into particularly troublesome joints from time to time.

About DMARDs

- All DMARDs require a long time to take effect—eight to twelve weeks—and need to be taken long term for the effect to be maintained. In other words, you do not stop taking them as soon as you feel better!

- Not all DMARDs are effective in all individuals, so if the first one that you try does not help, your rheumatologist may suggest you try a different one, or perhaps a combination of drugs.

- All DMARDs have side effects but, in general, these can be picked up very early by blood tests and urine tests, before any harm is done. So anyone taking these drugs will need to have regular tests to monitor for problems. You should be given a booklet by your rheumatologist or pharmacist to record the results of these tests.

There is more about this and other types of treatment in the chapter starting on page 71.

The outlook

If the condition is not treated, rheumatoid arthritis sufferers experience relapses (flares) and remissions. Flares may be triggered by illness, such as influenza, or even by stress, such as a bereavement. If the flares are frequent and severe, then damage to joints accumulates and they may be destroyed.

Fortunately, severe disease affecting the joints and other body tissues is rare. When first given the diagnosis, many people are shocked and upset and a common question is "Will I be in a wheelchair, doctor?"

They fear that rheumatoid arthritis automatically means immobility, disability, and dependency. This is no longer true.

Many sufferers have only mild arthritis and symptoms of pain and stiffness are kept at bay with pills and exercise. Even those with more extensive problems can, with the right help, lead almost normal lives with jobs and families. There is more about this and other types of treatment in the chapter starting on page 71.

KEY POINTS

- Rheumatoid arthritis causes joints to become inflamed—it is very different from osteoarthritis

- A lot of help is available for people with rheumatoid arthritis, although their care often requires the participation of a number of medical specialists and other healthcare professionals

Gout

Who gets gout?

There is a popular belief that only middle-aged, overweight men who eat and drink too much suffer from gout. This is a myth—gout can attack young men in their twenties and also women, although it is very unusual in women and occurs mainly after menopause. Gout may affect as many as 5 to 7 out of 1,000 men and 1 out of every 1,000 women in the United States.

What's happening?

An attack of gout is caused when uric acid crystals suddenly form inside a joint, causing intense inflammation with pain, redness, and swelling. Uric acid is produced when purines, which are chemicals present within all living cells, are broken down. Purines are produced by the body itself and are also found in many foods. People prone to gout have an inherited tendency to produce a lot of uric acid. High levels accumulate in the bloodstream and are deposited in the body's tissues.

Common sites are the joints, the kidneys, and the skin covering the tops of the ears, hands, and elbows. If the kidneys are affected, then they do not work as well as they should at excreting the uric acid in the urine and the levels become even higher. Uric acid deposits under the skin appear as whitish lumps, called "tophi." They may ulcerate and discharge material that looks like toothpaste. It is not always clear what causes the uric acid suddenly to form crystals in the joints and cause inflammation, but a common trigger is minor injury to the joint.

Symptoms

A typical attack of gout is easily recognizable (see below).

What happens during an attack of gout

- At first, there is only minor discomfort but, within a matter of hours, the joint is swollen, hot, red, and extremely painful.

- The pain is so severe that wearing shoes is out of the question, and you may not even be able to bear the touch of a bedsheet.

- Even with no treatment, the attack subsides completely within a few days, and always within a week.

- Attacks may recur, although sometimes not until months or years later.

- In 70 percent of people, the joint at the base of the big toe is the first joint, and often the only joint, to be affected, although symptoms can develop in any joint.

Diagnosis

Often your doctor will be able to recognize that you have gout from your symptoms and the appearance of the affected joint. You will need to have blood tests to measure the amount of uric acid in your bloodstream and to check whether your kidneys have been affected. A sample of fluid may sometimes be taken from an acutely inflamed joint, using a fine needle and syringe.

Examination of the fluid under a special polarizing microscope will show crystals of uric acid. This test will distinguish between gout and a condition known as "pseudogout." In pseudogout, the symptoms of an acute attack may mimic gout but the crystals responsible are calcium pyrophosphate. Pseudogout occurs in elderly people with osteoarthritis and is not usually inherited.

Treatment

Nonsteroidal anti-inflammatory drugs are very effective and can shorten an attack if they are taken right at the beginning. Before these drugs became available, the traditional treatment for an attack of gout was a drug called colchicine, derived from the autumn crocus.

Colchicine is still used and it is also very effective, although it can cause troublesome diarrhea in some people. In fact, both anti-inflammatory drugs and colchicine are so effective if taken early that people who have frequent attacks of gout are well advised to keep a supply in the medicine cabinet, so they can take it at the first sign of trouble.

Looking ahead

If you still get frequent attacks (e.g. more than three times a year) despite these measures, your doctor may

Diagnosing gout as a cause of joint pain

An attack of gout is caused by uric acid suddenly forming crystals within a joint, causing intense inflammation with pain, redness and swelling.

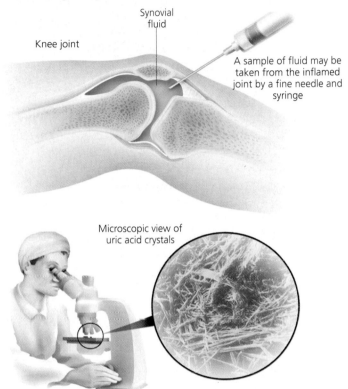

Synovial fluid

Knee joint

A sample of fluid may be taken from the inflamed joint by a fine needle and syringe

Microscopic view of uric acid crystals

suggest that you take drugs to lower the level of uric acid in your body. The main one is allopurinol which, taken daily as tablets, blocks the chemical pathway leading to uric acid production.

The uric acid deposits in the body tissues are then slowly removed into the urine and leave the body. This

Help yourself to avoid gout attacks

- Drink plenty of clear fluids (such as water), at least 8 to 10 glasses a day, especially in hot weather and when you're on vacation, because an attack is more likely if you become dehydrated.

- Reduce your weight so that it is within the normal range for your height (see page 108).

- Keep your alcohol consumption within recommended levels—28 units a week for a man and 21 for a woman. A unit is half a bottle of beer, a small glass of wine, or a single shot of hard liquor.

- Cut down on food and drink containing high levels of purines; these include high-protein foods such as red meats, organ meats (especially liver and kidneys), sardines, and anchovies. It is better to eat meals based around complex carbohydrates, such as pasta. If you are concerned about what you should be eating, ask to see a dietician.

- Avoid taking aspirin, which stops the kidneys from excreting uric acid; take acetaminophen instead for minor aches and pains.

effect takes place slowly, and you will still be prone to attacks of gout while the level of uric acid in your body remains high. Other drugs, less commonly used, work by making the kidneys more effective at excreting uric acid.

When you first start taking any of these long-term treatments, there is a temporarily increased risk of having an attack of gout, so you will usually be advised to take an anti-inflammatory drug at the same time for the first three months. Once you are on the long-term preventive treatment, you will probably have to continue with it indefinitely.

KEY POINTS

- Gout attacks are very painful but they disappear within a few days, even without treatment

- If attacks are frequent, then you may need to take medication every day to reduce the level of uric acid in your body

Other forms of inflammatory arthritis

Osteoarthritis, rheumatoid arthritis, and gout are the most common forms of arthritis but there are several other types that are also important, although they are much rarer. Some of these forms of arthritis develop in people with other conditions—the arthritis may be a major part of the disease or be a relatively minor problem. In these forms of arthritis, the joints are inflamed, that is, like rheumatoid arthritis, they are forms of inflammatory arthritis.

Ankylosing spondylitis
This condition causes inflammation of the joints in the spine, including the sacroiliac joints which link the spine to the pelvis, and the hips are also sometimes affected. It is three times more common in men than in women and it usually develops between the ages of 20 and 40. The risk is 10 to 20 times higher for those who have a parent, brother, or sister with the condition.

Ankylosing spondylitis is closely linked with an inherited factor known as tissue type HLA-B27. Only about 8 percent of the population have HLA-B27, but 95 percent of ankylosing spondylitis sufferers carry this tissue type.

Symptoms of ankylosing spondylitis

The main symptom is pain and stiffness in the lower back and hips, which is much worse in the mornings when it often lasts for several hours. The spine loosens up with activity and exercise but the stiffness recurs the following morning. Without treatment, the stiffness may spread to involve the whole spine, including the neck.

A program of daily exercises and regular review by a physiotherapist are vital to maintain the flexibility of the spine. Without regular exercise, the spine, over time, becomes curved and fixed. Drugs can ease the pain and the subjective feeling of stiffness, but they cannot take the place of exercise in maintaining movement.

Occasionally, other joints may be affected, and pain under the heel (plantar fasciitis, see page 68) can be troublesome. Sufferers may occasionally develop inflammation of the eye with redness, painful watering, and blurred vision. This requires urgent treatment from an ophthalmologist.

A number of other conditions are similar to ankylosing spondylitis. The whole group is known medically as "spondyloarthritis." These other conditions are described below.

Reactive arthritis (sometimes called Reiter's syndrome)

This develops in some people after an infection of the bowel or urogenital system. A small number of joints, usually a knee, or an ankle, or both, become very swollen and painful. The joints are not infected but the inflammation develops as a result of the body's reaction to the infection—hence the term "reactive arthritis." Back pain, eye inflammation, and a rash on the soles of the feet can also occur.

Inflammatory bowel disease, particularly ulcerative colitis

This can occasionally cause joint inflammation, in a pattern similar to ankylosing spondylitis but also affecting large joints such as hips, knees, or ankles.

Psoriatic arthritis

Psoriasis is a very common skin condition which affects about two percent of the population. A small proportion of these—less than 10 percent—develop inflammatory arthritis. The joint problems may develop even though the psoriasis is mild and, occasionally, they may appear before any skin changes.

On the other hand, psoriasis sufferers with severe skin disease may never have joint problems. Psoriatic arthritis is a form of spondyloarthritis but in severe cases it can be difficult to distinguish it from rheumatoid arthritis as it often affects the small joints of the hands and feet, as well as the large joints.

Symptoms of psoriatic arthritis

Unlike rheumatoid arthritis, psoriatic arthritis may occur unevenly. In other words, one hand may be affected but not the other. Eight out of ten people with psoriatic arthritis will notice that psoriasis affects their nails, so that they become pitted and chalky.

Around a third of people experience lower back pain as a result of inflammation in their sacroiliac joints, something that rarely happens in rheumatoid arthritis. Mild cases are treated with exercise and anti-inflammatory drugs. For severe cases, the drug treatment is similar to that for rheumatoid arthritis (see page 71).

Arthritis in children

Children may develop painful and swollen joints, usually after a viral infection or an injury, and the condition usually settles quickly. Arthritis that lasts for more than 12 weeks is unusual and may be caused by chronic inflammation. This condition is called "juvenile chronic arthritis" and in the United States has been found to affect 9 to 13 of every 100,000 children. The number of joints affected varies from one individual to another. Some children develop eye inflammation and some may be ill with a fever and a rash.

All children with arthritis need specialized care, and the health professionals, working together with parents and teachers, can ensure that the child can live as normal a life as possible.

Many children grow out of the condition in a few years, but a few have persistent problems as they grow up and a small number develop an adult form of the condition.

KEY POINTS

- There are several types of inflammatory arthritis—rheumatoid arthritis is the most common

- Children and young people can develop inflammatory arthritis and their care should involve specialized physicians and other healthcare professionals

Other inflammatory conditions

Some other conditions, unrelated to spondyloarthritis, can cause inflammation associated with mild arthritis. The inflammation is more widespread and, as well as the joints, it affects tissues elsewhere in the body. The Arthritis Foundation (see Useful addresses on page 112) publishes free information leaflets about all of these conditions.

Systemic lupus erythematosus

Systemic lupus erythematosus (SLE or lupus) belongs to a group of conditions called "connective tissue diseases" (connective tissue supports and connects other body parts). SLE is similar to rheumatoid arthritis in that it is an autoimmune disease (see page 22) but it is much rarer and the arthritis is usually much less severe. Around 90 percent of those affected are young women between the ages of 20 and 40, and African-American women are particularly susceptible.

Symptoms of SLE

- Painful, swollen joints, particularly in the hands
- Feeling generally unwell and feverish
- Rash on the face, particularly in response to sunlight
- Thinning of the hair.

Most people with SLE have a mild form that comes and goes, affecting only their joints and skin, and causing mild anemia. A few develop severe inflammation of the internal organs, such as the kidneys, lungs, and nervous system, and some women suffer repeated miscarriages. SLE responds very well to steroids but, in cases of severe disease, other drugs that suppress the immune system may also be needed.

Polymyositis

Polymyositis is also a connective tissue disorder, rarer than SLE. It mainly affects the muscles which become inflamed and very weak. In the related condition of dermatomyositis, the skin is also affected. Both conditions respond to steroids that may need to be used in large doses for a while.

Polymyalgia rheumatica

Polymyalgia rheumatica (PMR) is quite a common condition. It affects older people and is very rare in anyone younger than 50. It is not related to the connective tissue diseases.

"Polymyalgia" literally means "pain in many muscles" but the condition appears to result from inflammation in the joints of the shoulder girdle and pelvic girdle, rather than in the muscles.

Symptoms of PMR

- Severe pain and stiffness around the shoulders and hips, that is noticeably much worse in the mornings
- Difficulty turning over in bed at night without help
- Feeling generally unwell and tired, sometimes feverish
- Loss of weight
- Depression.

Diagnosis of PMR

Your doctor will often be able to diagnose the condition from the symptoms you describe and the results of a blood test to measure the erythrocyte sedimentation rate (ESR). The ESR is usually very high in polymyalgia (see page 11), indicating the presence of inflammation.

Treatment of PMR

Steroids taken by mouth or by injection have a dramatic effect and within 24 hours you should feel almost back to normal. The steroids should not be stopped too quickly as you may need to be treated for many months (occasionally, for several years) to fully eliminate the discomfort, and decrease the likelihood that the symptoms may reappear.

For more about treatments see "Treating arthritis and rheumatism" on page 71.

KEY POINTS

■ Some rare conditions cause inflammation in many areas of the body, including the joints; these are best treated with steroids, which are powerful anti-inflammatory drugs

Non-inflammatory conditions

Fibromyalgia

Fibromyalgia is often confused with polymyalgia (see page 42) but in fibromyalgia there is no sign of inflammation. People with fibromyalgia are often worried that they have arthritis or some other serious disease but this is rarely the case. The results of blood tests and X-rays are normal.

Most people with fibromyalgia are women in their middle years. In some cases the symptoms seem to be triggered by bereavement or stress and they are often associated with poor sleep (see below). It can be difficult to decide whether the chronic pain of the condition led to the symptoms of tiredness, fatigue, and poor sleep, or whether insufficient sleep or poor quality sleep is actually the root cause of the problem.

Symptoms of fibromyalgia

- Widespread pain and tenderness, particularly across the shoulders, back, elbows, and knees

- Although the joints and soft tissues are tender, they are not swollen
- The muscles and joints may feel stiff in the mornings but this disappears quickly after getting up
- Low spirits or depression
- Poor sleep
- Lack of energy.

Treatment

The doctor may prescribe medication to lift depression and help you to sleep more soundly if necessary. Remaining as active and mobile as possible will help. If you rest a lot, you may feel worse as you will become "deconditioned" and more tired and your muscles will become weaker and more susceptible to injury. Regular exercise can also help clear your mind and improve the quality of your sleep. You can help yourself with other simple lifestyle changes (see box below) in addition to any treatment provided by your physicians.

Self-help tips for fibromyalgia

- Don't drink coffee or other caffeine-containing drinks in the evening because they may disturb your sleep
- Consider relaxation classes
- Try to deal with any major sources of stress in your daily life
- Keep as active as possible, and consider taking up some gentle, regular exercise such as swimming or brisk walking

Hypermobility

This is not actually a disease but it may be a cause of very painful joints in young people. People come in all shapes and sizes and there is a similar variation in joint flexibility. Some people normally have rather stiff joints whereas, at the other extreme, some have very supple, mobile joints and are often called "double-jointed." If you are one of these people, you may be able to bend over with your knees straight and put your hands flat on the floor in front of you when most of us struggle just to touch our toes. Your elbows and knees may bend backward and your fingers may turn up when you hold them outstretched. If you can do this, you may have "hypermobility syndrome."

Hypermobility represents the supple end of the normal spectrum of joint mobility. A small number of people with extremely mobile joints suffer recurrent dislocations and their joints are easily damaged but most people with hypermobility have it in a mild form. Very supple joints are easily strained by everyday activities and people with painful, hypermobile joints

Self-help tips for hypermobile joints

- Take care not to strain your joints
- Exercise regularly to build up your muscles—well-toned muscles will help to support your joints and protect them from strain
- Avoid exercises or activities that overstretch the joints, such as ballet and gymnastics
- Most important of all, resist the temptation to perform "party tricks" to show off your mobile joints

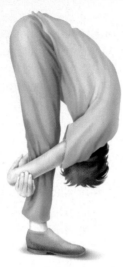

Hypermobility represents the supple end of the normal spectrum of joint mobility.

may worry that they have arthritis although this is unlikely to be the case. A few simple measures will help to keep the pain under control (see page 47).

Neck and back problems
Back pain

Lower back pain, or lumbago, is very common: 80 percent of the population experience it at some time in their lives. Most back pain is "nonspecific" or "mechanical"—in other words, it results from some minor physical problem in the complex structure of the back, such as a strained muscle, ligament, or tendon, which will heal on its own in time. Serious causes of back pain are very rare indeed. Surprisingly, the severity of the pain is not a good guide to the seriousness of the cause and, in fact, the most severe pains are usually nonspecific and should heal in their own time.

Correcting poor posture, taking care with lifting and carrying, and performing regular exercise can all help. Much useful information about the spine can be found in the book *Understanding Back Pain* in the Family Doctor series.

Sciatica

Sometimes pain is felt in one of the legs as well as in the back. Sciatica, which is caused by pressure on a nerve by a disk in the spine, is one cause and the leg pain may be accompanied by tingling, pins-and-needles or numbness. This is often referred to as a "slipped disk." A more correct name is "prolapsed disk" or "ruptured disk." Disks are filled with a jelly which acts as a cushion between the bones of the spinal column. When a disk ruptures or tears, some of this jelly squirts out and can irritate a nearby nerve, causing severe pain down the leg (see diagram on page 50).

Treatment

With painkillers, a few days' rest, and then gentle exercise and physiotherapy, the tear heals, the disk material is absorbed, and the pressure on the nerve is relieved. Most people are completely cured in a few weeks, but in a very few, the symptoms do not disappear with painkillers and physiotherapy and surgery may be needed to remove the disk material.

Neck pain

Pain in the neck is probably as common as pain in the back and often has similar causes, although a ruptured disk is much less common in the neck than in the lower back. Poor posture is a common culprit. Many people

Back pain caused by prolapsed disc

Sometimes pain is felt in one of the legs as well as in the back. This may be caused by a prolapsed disc in the spine.

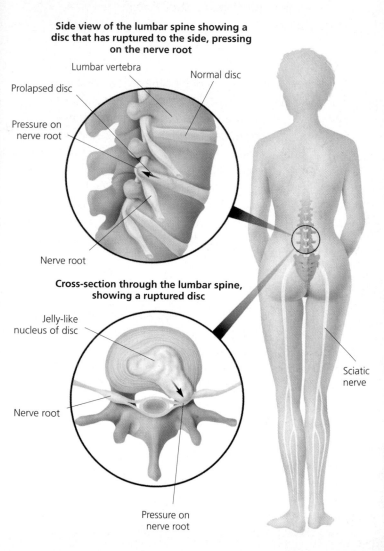

Side view of the lumbar spine showing a disc that has ruptured to the side, pressing on the nerve root

Lumbar vertebra

Normal disc

Prolapsed disc

Pressure on nerve root

Nerve root

Cross-section through the lumbar spine, showing a ruptured disc

Jelly-like nucleus of disc

Nerve root

Pressure on nerve root

Sciatic nerve

hunch their shoulders and allow the head to poke forward. The head is very heavy (as heavy as a bucket of water) and, to stop the head from flopping onto the chest, the muscles at the back of the neck have to work hard to hold the head up.

Eventually, this chronic contraction, or tension, causes aching pain and stiffness in the trapezius muscles across the shoulders, and up the neck to the back of the head. It can even cause severe headaches (tension headaches) felt across the forehead and behind the eyes.

Treatment
Treatment involves understanding the problem, correcting the posture, and performing regular simple exercises to loosen the muscles and keep the neck supple.

Arthritis of the spine
Degenerative arthritis, or spondylosis, of the spine is extremely common. If an X-ray were taken of the spine of everyone over the age of 50, almost all of them would show degenerative changes. But not all of these people have back pain and, of those who do, the pain often comes and goes. So there is no clear relationship between X-ray changes and symptoms. Regardless of whether there are degenerative changes on the X-ray, most episodes of back pain will get better with painkillers and a few days' rest, followed by gentle exercise and then getting back to normal activities. But if the back pain lasts longer than a week and you find it difficult to get back to work, then you should consult your doctor.

Another form of arthritis that affects the spine is ankylosing spondylitis. This is a rare form of inflammatory arthritis and it has been described earlier (see page 36).

Osteoporosis

In older people, especially women, pain in the upper back may be the result of osteoporosis ("thinning of the bones'). Everyone loses calcium from their bones as they get older, especially women after menopause. The process is usually very slow, but there may come a point when the bones have lost so much calcium that they are thin and prone to fracture. The vertebrae in the upper back may become distorted so that the back becomes very rounded ("widow's hump"). There may be chronic pain or episodes of acute pain, when a single bone collapses slightly. If you think you may have osteoporosis, consult your doctor.

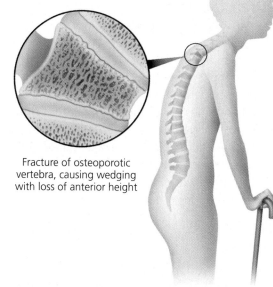

Fracture of osteoporotic
vertebra, causing wedging
with loss of anterior height

In osteoporosis, the bones become thinner and weaker.
Vertebrae may collapse, causing the back to become rounded.

Treatments are now available that can slow down the loss of calcium from the bones and even make them a little stronger. You can help by giving up smoking, making sure your diet contains plenty of calcium and taking regular exercise—even a brisk walk for half an hour three times a week can make a difference.

Much more detailed information about osteoporosis is contained in the book *Understanding Osteoporosis* in the Family Doctor series, or can be obtained from the National Osteoporosis Foundation (see Useful addresses, page 112).

Problems in and around individual joints

"Soft-tissue rheumatism" is the term used to describe a group of painful conditions that are caused by problems with the soft tissues around joints, rather than problems with the joints themselves. Tendons, which join muscles to bone, ligaments, which join bones together, and bursas can all be responsible.

The general principles of treatment of these conditions involve steroid injections to ease the pain and decrease the inflammation in the acute phase, a splint to rest the painful area, and, most important of all, recognizing what activity caused the problem and either avoiding the activity altogether or changing the way that it is performed. If this aspect of the treatment is neglected, then there is a risk that the problem will recur. Many sports injuries fall into this category.

Shoulder pain

Pain felt around the shoulder can sometimes be caused by neck problems. This is particularly true if the pain is felt on top of the shoulder in the large trapezius muscle that runs between the shoulder joint and the neck.

Pain arising from the shoulder joint itself is often felt in the upper arm rather than over the point of the shoulder. Common causes are frozen shoulder (also known as "adhesive capsulitis") and tendonitis.

Frozen shoulder

This mainly affects older people and is rare under the age of 50. The symptoms usually begin suddenly and may result from a minor injury, such as a knock or a fall, although the injury may be so minor as to be forgotten. Occasionally, frozen shoulder can follow an attack of shingles or even a heart attack.

We do not know what causes frozen shoulder but we know that the capsule surrounding the joint becomes thickened and inflamed, causing pain. The inflamed capsule is "sticky" and adhesions form between the capsule and the bones, restricting the movement of the joint.

Symptoms of frozen shoulder

- Constant pain which can be very severe, even when the shoulder is held still.
- Difficulty sleeping because of the pain—it may also be impossible to lie on the affected side.
- Severe stiffness, which may make it very difficult to reach up to a shelf or into a back pocket or, in some cases, to move the joint at all.

Treatment

Even without treatment, the pain of a frozen shoulder will usually ease and disappear within 18 months, but most people don't want to wait that long! When the shoulder is intensely painful, the most effective treatment is steroid injection into the joint. This relieves the pain, although sometimes more than one injection is needed.

The other, equally important, aspect of treatment is regular exercise to bring back the range of motion and prevent the shoulder from becoming stiff and stuck once the pain has gone.

When performing the exercises described in the box below, don't stretch or move beyond the point where you feel slight pain. Forcing your shoulder through a wider range of movement will just make the problem worse. But with careful attention to regular exercise,

Exercises for frozen shoulder

- Stand up and lean your trunk slightly over toward the side of the affected shoulder, so that your arm hangs away from your body. Swing the arm gently backward and forward, keeping your elbow straight, and avoid shrugging your shoulder as you swing. Swing backward and forward 10 times and repeat the whole exercise several times a day.

- Lean forward and gently swing your arm from side to side across your body, moving the shoulder joint in a different direction, then swing the arm in a circular movement. As the shoulder becomes freer, you will find that you can swing farther and farther and in ever wider circles.

- Reach behind your waist with your good arm and grasp the wrist of the arm with the frozen shoulder. Gently pull the arm behind your back, being careful not to force the movement.

you should regain useful movement in your shoulder, although it may always remain slightly restricted compared with your normal side.

Shoulder tendonitis

Inflammation of the tendons or the sheaths containing them is a common cause of shoulder pain. A normal shoulder has an enormous range of motion—you can raise your arms up above your head, bring them out to the sides, and swing them up behind your back. This is a legacy from our evolutionary ancestors who needed this range of motion to swing through trees. Unfortunately, it means that the tendons of the shoulder are easily damaged and subject to wear. They can fray and bleed a little, leading to inflammation. This causes pain that is always worse when the shoulder is moved and less severe at rest.

Treatment

Injection of a steroid into the area around the inflamed tendon can be very effective. After a couple of days, you can start on a gentle program of exercise to restore normal movement to your shoulder. The exercises are likely to be similar to those for frozen shoulder (see page 55), but your doctor or physiotherapist will explain just what you need to do.

Once the pain has eased, you must resist the temptation to perform heavy lifting and you should pace any work that is heavy on the shoulders, such as cleaning windows, digging, or using a vacuum cleaner.

You should also beware the "perils of the plastic shopping bag"! Plastic shopping bags are very strong and some have small handles. They can be loaded with

Anatomy of the shoulder joint

In shoulder tendonitis, the tendons are damaged and in frozen shoulder the capsule is affected.

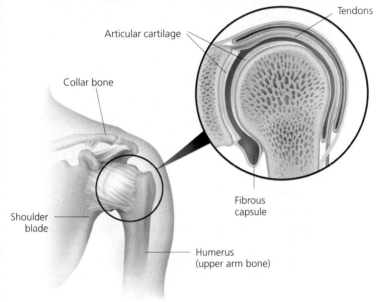

Tendons

Articular cartilage

Collar bone

Fibrous capsule

Shoulder blade

Humerus (upper arm bone)

heavy shopping and the small handles mean that the bags have to be carried with the arms held vertically downward. The weight drags on the elbows and shoulders and also the neck, straining the tissues and causing pain.

Heavy shopping should ideally be carried in a shopping cart. If this is not possible (carts can be difficult to load into a car or on public transportation), then small amounts of shopping can be placed in a stiff basket with a wide handle, carried over the forearm close to the elbow. Most of the weight of the basket can then be carried on the hip, avoiding undue strain on the arms.

Tennis elbow and golfer's elbow

These conditions cause pain at the points at which the tendon attaches to the bone around the elbow. Tennis elbow causes pain on the outer side of the elbow, at the point where the extensor muscles on the outer side of the forearm are attached (see diagram below). These muscles bend the wrist backward and straighten the fingers. Golfer's elbow is much less common and causes pain on the inner side of the elbow, at the attachment of the flexor muscles that bend the wrist forward and flex the fingers.

Both conditions were first described in athletes but most sufferers develop them as a result of everyday activities, such as repeated heavy lifting, pushing, and pulling. Sometimes a single episode of awkward lifting, such as lifting a heavy suitcase down from an overhead locker, may be the trigger. The lifting need not be heavy: office workers who repeatedly pull files from tight, over-stuffed cabinets are also at risk.

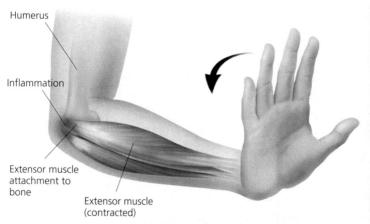

Humerus

Inflammation

Extensor muscle attachment to bone

Extensor muscle (contracted)

Right arm seen from the right side. When the extensor muscle contracts, to bend the wrist back, the muscle pulls on the bone. This causes pain if the area is inflamed, as in "tennis elbow."

Treatment

A steroid injection into the painful area is usually helpful. Physiotherapy may also be beneficial. But most important is to determine what caused the problem in the first place and avoid the activity in future, otherwise the symptoms may recur and can become chronic.

Overuse syndrome (repetitive strain injury, RSI)

There has been much discussion in the law courts (where sufferers have claimed compensation from their employers) as to whether this condition really exists, but most doctors agree that it does.

Like many other soft-tissue problems, this condition is triggered by misuse or overuse of the affected part of the body. It is also called "upper limb syndrome" and affects the neck, shoulders, arms, and hands of keyboard workers and other people who continually repeat the same tasks and movements in their work. In fact, people employed to pluck chickens were the first group in whom the condition was identified.

The pain is not confined to any one area but is most severe in the backs of the hands and forearms, and is clearly related to work. At first, it may begin only toward the end of a busy day. If left untreated, it can progress and then the time between starting work and developing the pain gets shorter.

In severe cases, there is some pain all the time, even when not at work, and normal daily activities outside work may also trigger pain.

Treatment

If the symptoms have been neglected and the condition has been allowed to become severe and chronic,

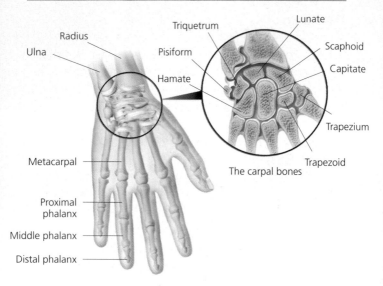

Radius
Ulna
Triquetrum
Pisiform
Hamate
Lunate
Scaphoid
Capitate
Trapezium
Trapezoid
The carpal bones

Metacarpal
Proximal phalanx
Middle phalanx
Distal phalanx

The wrist and hand contain very many bones.

treatment is difficult and not always successful. It is vital to act promptly as soon as you suspect that you may be developing problems. Look very carefully at the nature of your work and the design of your workstation. Physiotherapists and occupational therapists are experts in these assessments but there are a number of problem areas you can change yourself: see the self-help tips on pages 62–3. Discuss the situation with your employers and see your physician or the company's occupational health doctor, if there is one.

Although most cases of overuse syndrome occur as a result of practices at work, if you use a computer (or other equipment, such as a sewing machine) a lot at home, you can develop exactly the same problems. The principles of pacing, technique, proper positioning, and posture still apply. With careful attention to these principles, most people are able to continue with their work.

Carpal tunnel syndrome

In this very common condition, there is pressure on the median nerve as it passes through the wrist (see diagram on page 64). The bones of the wrist (the carpal bones) are arranged in a horseshoe shape. The free ends of the horseshoe are joined together by a tough piece of tissue, forming a narrow tunnel through which the median nerve passes.

Any swelling of the tissues in the area can cause pressure on the nerve and irritate it. Signals sent from the median nerve to the brain are interpreted as coming from the area supplied by this nerve—that is, from the hand (see below). Carpal tunnel syndrome can be caused by fluid retention, such as occurs in pregnancy or when the thyroid gland is underactive, or be a symptom of rheumatoid arthritis, but very often no underlying cause is identified.

Symptoms of carpal tunnel syndrome

- Numbness, tingling, or pain in the hand, worse in the thumb, index, and middle fingers.

- Symptoms are much worse during the night or first thing in the morning and may disappear completely during the day.

- Rubbing or shaking the hand eases the pain and tingling.

Treatment

The priority is to relieve the pressure on the nerve, which increases when your wrist is bent forward and reduces

Self-help tips to avoid RSI

- **Alternate your work.** Split it up and combine different tasks—instead of spending two whole days typing and then two days filing, alternate every few hours.

- **Take regular breaks.** If your job involves mainly one activity, such as using a computer, then it is vitally important that you take regular breaks. Every hour, stand up, stretch your legs, lift your arms above your head, and open and close your hands. Focus on distant objects through the window to rest your eyes. This takes only a couple of minutes but will make all the difference to how long you can work without discomfort.

- **Improve your technique.** If you're a keyboard worker and can't touch-type, it is worth learning to do so because this allows you to spread the work of typing over all your fingers and thumbs and means that you can hold your head up instead of looking down at the keyboard.

- **Make sure that your equipment and furniture are properly positioned.** You should have a height-adjustable chair on wheels, with a backrest and without arms so that you can sit close up to your desk. Your computer screen and keyboard should be placed directly in front of you—just a few inches to one side will place strain on your arms and neck. The screen should be slightly lower than your sight-line—any lower and you will hunch your shoulders and lean forward, any higher and you will crane your neck. All other equipment that you use regularly, such as the telephone, should be placed close to you so that you are not continually reaching across the desk.

Self-help tips to avoid RSI (contd)

- **Pay attention to your posture.** The best-designed equipment will do nothing for you if it is not used properly. Adjust the height of your chair so that your feet are comfortably placed on the floor or on a foot-rest and your forearms rest comfortably on the desk. Don't slouch in the chair but sit up straight, preserving the curve in your lower back. Sit close to your desk so that your hands rest on the keyboard without stretching your arms forward. Your shoulders should be relaxed, your upper arms should hang vertically downward and your forearms should be held at right angles when typing.

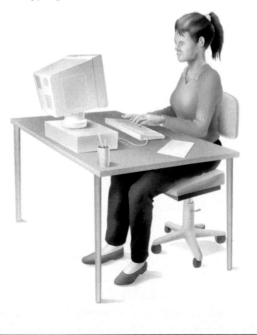

Carpal tunnel syndrome

Carpal tunnel syndrome is caused by pressure on the median nerve as it passes through the carpal tunnel – which is formed by the bones of the wrist and the ligaments over them.

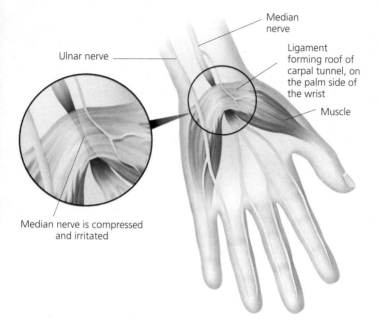

Median nerve

Ligament forming roof of carpal tunnel, on the palm side of the wrist

Muscle

Ulnar nerve

Median nerve is compressed and irritated

when it is bent backward. A simple splint worn around the wrist at night to stop it bending forward may be enough to solve the problem. These are generally available in well-stocked pharmacies and surgical supply stores or a physiotherapist can provide you with one. You can also help yourself by ensuring that your wrists are not bent forward when you are sitting with your hands in your lap or with your arms folded. If this does not work, then the injection of steroid into the carpal tunnel can shrink the tissues enough to relieve the pressure. If this is not effective either, a simple operation under local anesthetic will relieve the pressure on the nerve.

Thumb tendonitis (de Quervain's tenosynovitis)

In this condition, the pain arises from the tendons that work the thumb. Tendons run inside a lubricated sheath but, when they become inflamed, movement causes the surfaces to grate against each other (see diagram). The base of the thumb and the lower end of the forearm become painful, and the area may be tender and even swollen. Parents who lift their young children by holding them under the armpits are particularly prone to this complaint; so are restaurant

Thumb tendonitis

Tendons run inside a lubricated sheath but, when they become inflamed, movement causes the surfaces to grate against each other resulting in pain.

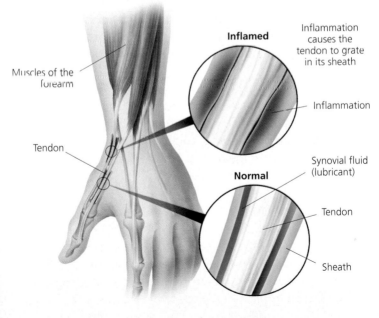

Muscles of the forearm

Inflamed

Inflammation causes the tendon to grate in its sheath

Inflammation

Tendon

Normal

Synovial fluid (lubricant)

Tendon

Sheath

staff who carry heavy plates of food in each hand with the weight balanced by the thumb.

Osteoarthritis of the joint at the base of the thumb, where it is attached to the wrist, can cause similar symptoms.

Treatment

Thumb tendonitis usually responds very well to a steroid injection into the sheath of the tendon together with a splint to rest the thumb. It is also very important to identify the activity that caused the problem and avoid it.

Trigger finger

Make a fist and then straighten your fingers. If one finger lags behind the others, at first refusing to straighten and then suddenly straightening with a "click," you have trigger finger. The condition is the result of a nodule that develops on the tendon as it runs through the palm of the hand. The nodule catches on the edge of the tendon sheath during movement.

Treatment

If the nodule is painless and does not affect the use of your hand, it is probably best left alone because it may settle by itself. If necessary, you can be given a steroid injection to shrink the nodule and free the tendon.

Knee pain

Most people have painful knees at some time in their lives. In older people, osteoarthritis is common but there are many other causes of knee pain, especially in younger people. The knee is subjected to considerable stresses, especially if you are very overweight. Some sports, such as football, skiing, tennis, soccer, and basketball, require your knees to rotate and bend and bear your weight at the same time, placing the knees under great strain.

All this means that the knees are susceptible to a wide range of injuries, often affecting the shock-absorbing cartilage pads within the joint and the many ligaments that hold the joint together (see diagram below). Many injuries will heal naturally but some may need splints or even surgery.

Anatomy of the knee

The bones of the knee are held together by strong ligaments.

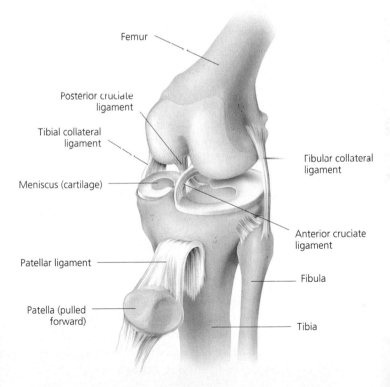

Femur

Posterior cruciate ligament

Tibial collateral ligament

Fibular collateral ligament

Meniscus (cartilage)

Anterior cruciate ligament

Patellar ligament

Fibula

Patella (pulled forward)

Tibia

Look after your knees

- Avoid squatting and kneeling, which strain the knees.
- Keep your weight down. If you are overweight, losing just a few pounds can help your pain and make all the difference to the strain on your knees.
- Avoid sitting in low, soft chairs. Getting out of them can be difficult if you have painful knees.
- Keep your thigh muscles strong with exercises (see page 94), especially if you participate in sports.
- Do not sleep with a pillow under your knees. It may feel comfortable but your knees can become permanently bent.

Pain under the heel

Pain in the sole of the foot, directly under the heel, is often caused by plantar fasciitis. This troublesome condition causes pain that is particularly severe when you first get out of bed in the morning but then eases a little as you continue to walk. The plantar fascia is a tough fibrous band, shaped like a triangle, which joins the ball of the foot with the heel bone. The strain and inflammation occur at the point where the fascia joins the heel bone. Sometimes, an extra bit of bone, known as a spur, may grow at this point.

Plantar fasciitis often affects people who are on their feet a lot in their work and those who are overweight, so good footwear and losing weight can help. It can also be a feature of some types of inflammatory arthritis (see page 37), but this is unusual.

In older people, pain under the heel can also be the result of thinning of the fat pad. There is normally a dense cushion of tissue, mostly fat, under the heel, which acts as a shock absorber when walking. This cushion may become thin as you get older and the heel bone is no longer so well protected. Well-fitting shoes with soft, sponge rubber soles and heels, perhaps with a soft insole as well, will protect the heels.

Treatment

Steroid injection often helps plantar fasciitis but, because the injection can be very painful, other options may be tried first. These include an anti-inflammatory drug, wearing heel cups made of dense, shock-absorbing foam inside your shoes, and strapping put on by a

Anatomy of the foot

Bones of the right foot seen from the left side. In plantar fasciitis there is pain and inflammation at the site where the plantar fascia ligament joins the heel bone.

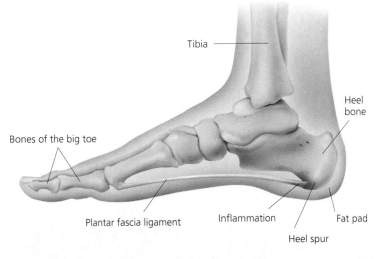

Tibia

Heel bone

Bones of the big toe

Plantar fascia ligament

Inflammation

Fat pad

Heel spur

physiotherapist or podiatrist. Losing weight, if you are overweight, and avoiding prolonged standing, can also help.

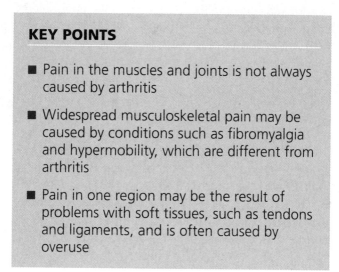

KEY POINTS

- Pain in the muscles and joints is not always caused by arthritis

- Widespread musculoskeletal pain may be caused by conditions such as fibromyalgia and hypermobility, which are different from arthritis

- Pain in one region may be the result of problems with soft tissues, such as tendons and ligaments, and is often caused by overuse

Treating arthritis and rheumatism

A multidisciplinary approach

Many people with locomotor problems will need more than one type of treatment—for example, drugs combined with physiotherapy and a program of exercise to rehabilitate joints and soft tissues. Brief details of treatments for specific conditions are given in the preceding chapters. This section covers the treatments that may be used for arthritis and soft-tissue rheumatism in general.

Drugs

Analgesics, or painkillers, and nonsteroidal anti-inflammatory drugs are the most important drugs in the treatment of arthritis and rheumatism. They are especially useful when the underlying cause of the symptoms cannot be cured.

Analgesics

Examples of analgesics (often called "simple analgesics" to distinguish them from anti-inflammatory drugs, which also act as painkillers) are acetaminophen and codeine. Combinations of the two are also available without prescription under different trade names but the others are prescription-only drugs.

Many of these medications, except acetaminophen, can cause drowsiness and constipation.

Simple analgesics relieve pain but they do not have any anti-inflammatory action so they have little effect on stiffness and swelling.

Anti-inflammatory drugs

Non-steroidal anti-inflammatory drugs (NSAIDs— pronounced "en-seds") can often be very helpful when simple analgesics fail to relieve symptoms. They are so-called because they reduce inflammation, which steroids also do, but they are completely different from steroids in the way that they work and in their potential side effects. NSAIDs are particularly effective in combating the stiffness and swelling that are caused by inflammation, as well as the pain.

The oldest anti-inflammatory drug is aspirin. Unfortunately, it needs to be given in large doses for it to have an anti-inflammatory effect (as distinct from a painkilling effect) and in large doses it has a high risk of producing side effects, especially on the stomach. It has been superseded by more modern drugs with fewer side effects, such as ibuprofen, diclofenac, and naproxen.

Guidelines for using simple analgesics

- Start with acetaminophen, which is the simplest, safest, and most inexpensive analgesic, and which, if taken correctly, is very effective.

- Always follow the instructions on the packaging and never exceed the recommended dose—all drugs are dangerous if you take too many, including acetaminophen.

- If you have constant or frequent pain, take painkillers regularly throughout the day, rather than waiting until the pain becomes really troublesome.

- If you have a lot of pain at night, take your painkillers half an hour before bedtime.

- If you are planning a shopping trip or some other activity that you know will worsen your pain, take your painkillers half an hour before you set out.

- If you find that the painkillers you are taking are not strong enough or you are taking them continuously, consult your doctor as there may be better pain-relieving strategies which could reduce your need for analgesics. Keep a record of how long each package or bottle lasts you so that your doctor knows how many you've been taking.

REMEMBER: Many proprietary cold and flu treatments contain acetaminophen, and there is a risk of an accidental overdose if you are already taking acetaminophen (e.g. Tylenol) regularly for pain relief.

NSAIDs and the stomach

Why do NSAIDs cause stomach irritation? All NSAIDs work by blocking the production of prostaglandins in the tissues. Prostaglandins are chemicals released by cells at the site of an injury or damage caused by disease. They increase the flow of blood to the inflamed area, making it red and hot, and cause the blood vessels to become "leaky," causing the area to become swollen.

Unfortunately, blocking prostaglandin production has negative as well as positive effects. This is because other types of prostaglandins, not involved in disease, play an important part in protecting the stomach lining from being damaged by its own digestive juices and acid. Unfortunately, NSAIDs block all prostaglandins, including the stomach protectors. This is why side effects such as indigestion, ulcers, and bleeding from the stomach wall can all occur in people who take NSAIDs.

COX-2 inhibitors

Newer NSAIDs (known as selective COX-2 or cyclo-oxygenase inhibitors), such as celecoxib (Celebrex) appear to act in a specific way and their blocking effect is concentrated on the inflammatory prostaglandins rather than the protective ones (they reduce prostaglandin production at sites of pain and inflammation without affecting production in the stomach). In theory, these drugs look promising but it is not yet clear what their long-term side effects might be.

A related drug, rofecoxib (Vioxx), was taken off the market recently because of unexpected side effects (an increase in the risk of heart attacks).

As a result of these concerns COX-2 inhibitors should be avoided by people who have heart disease or

NSAIDs and stomach ulcers

Some anti-arthritis drugs (NSAIDs) can interfere with the digestive system.

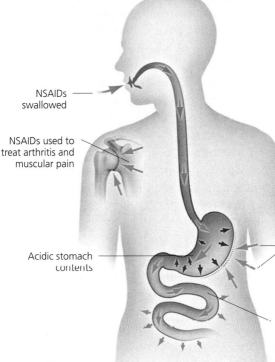

NSAIDs swallowed

NSAIDs used to treat arthritis and muscular pain

Acidic stomach contents

NSAIDs weaken the protective layer of the stomach lining, increasing the likelihood of peptic ulcers

NSAIDs are absorbed in the intestine, into the blood, and are carried to all parts of the body

vascular disease (diseases of blood vessels or "hardening of the arteries").

Currently, it has not been determined that the other COX-2 inhibitors (or indeed other non-selective NSAIDs) have the same level of risk as rofecoxib (Vioxx).

However, it has become clear that COX-2 inhibitors have fewer gastrointestinal effects than NSAIDs, in particular the incidence of life-threatening ulcer complications such as bleeding and perforation.

At present, this group of drugs is likely to be prescribed for you only if you develop gastric problems while on NSAIDs or have had ulcers in the past, and if you do not have heart disease or vascular disease.

As a rule, NSAIDs offer most benefit to people with a form of inflammatory arthritis, such as rheumatoid arthritis, or who have developed an acute inflammation, such as gout. People with osteoarthritis and the soft-tissue problems described in the preceding chapter should begin with simple analgesics, which have fewer side effects, and change to an NSAID, for the shortest possible time, only if the analgesic does not work.

Steroids

Steroids are produced naturally by the body. There are many different types and they act in many different ways. Many steroids can now be manufactured in the form of pills and injections, and they are prescribed by doctors to treat a variety of conditions.

People often become worried when their doctor says that they need steroids. They have heard a lot about side effects and also about the abuse of steroids by some athletes and body-builders. But the steroids used in arthritis are quite different from those abused in sports. The steroids used to treat arthritis are powerful anti-inflammatory drugs and they are very effective in controlling swelling, stiffness, and pain. There is even some evidence from research that, in certain circumstances, they can reduce the damage done to joints by rheumatoid arthritis.

Guidelines for using anti-inflammatory drugs (NSAIDs)

- Ibuprofen is among the most widely available NSAID with the fewest side effects, so, unless your doctor advises otherwise, you may wish to start with ibuprofen.

- Ibuprofen is available over the counter in a number of branded formulas but the unbranded or "generic" version may be cheaper and just as effective.

- If an NSAID reduces stiffness and swelling but you still have some pain, then also taking a simple analgesic, such as paracetamol, can be helpful. It is quite safe to do this, as the two drugs work in different ways and do not interact.

- All NSAIDs must be taken with food and *never* on an empty stomach and, if you get a stomach upset, you must stop taking them. This is because they can irritate the lining of the stomach, causing indigestion and even ulcers and bleeding. All NSAIDs have this side effect to some extent, although only a minority of people who take them suffer from it.

- If you are elderly or if you have had an ulcer in the past, you are more susceptible to stomach irritation. You should consult your doctor before you take an NSAID. You may be given a combination treatment of an NSAID together with a drug to protect the stomach.

- If you have asthma, you need to be aware that occasionally aspirin and other NSAIDs may bring on an attack.

continues

Guidelines for using anti-inflammatory drugs (NSAIDs) (contd)

- Some NSAIDs are also available in the form of a gel that is massaged into the painful area. This can help pain that arises from the tissues near the surface of the skin, but is of little help in the pain of arthritis because the joints are too deep for the drug to penetrate to them.

Steroids can be taken in a variety of ways:

- In high doses for short periods to treat a flare in conditions such as systemic lupus erythematosus. The steroids may be given by mouth or, in severe cases, in a hospital by direct injection into a vein.

- By single injection into the buttock muscle. This method is often used in people with rheumatoid arthritis who have just started taking drugs to control the arthritis long term. The steroid injection can tide them over while their drugs take effect—usually several weeks.

- In lower doses taken by mouth over the long term to keep inflammation under control in conditions such as polymyalgia rheumatica.

- Injected directly into a problem area such as an inflamed joint, tendon sheath, or other soft tissue.

Possible side effects of steroids

Like all drugs, steroids can have side effects. But despite the long list of side effects, steroids are powerful, effective drugs which are invaluable if used wisely (see "Guidelines," page 79). For example, when polymyalgia sufferers start taking steroids, they feel that they have been given a new lease on life.

The possible side effects of long-term steroids

- Weight gain caused by an increase in appetite and retention of fluid
- Raised blood pressure
- Increased risk of developing diabetes and poor control of blood sugar levels in people who already have diabetes
- Increased susceptibility to infections
- Increased risk of stomach ulcers and bleeding
- Increased risk of developing osteoporosis
- Thinning of the skin and slow healing of cuts and grazes

Guidelines for taking long-term steroids

- Steroid treatment should always be prescribed and supervised by a doctor. Never adjust the dose except on the advice of a doctor
- You may wish to carry a card or wear a bracelet that indicates that you are receiving ongoing treatment with steroids and you should have the card with you or wear the bracelet at all times
- If you are taken ill or injured, you must tell the doctor treating you that you take steroids and show him or her your card or bracelet
- Steroid pills should be taken in the early morning, when the levels of natural steroids are at their peak. This causes less suppression of the adrenal glands
- Instead of a dose every day, your doctor may suggest that you take double the dose on alternate days. This also can reduce the effect on the adrenal glands.

Unfortunately, it is not always possible to do this as some people find that their symptoms are much worse on the non-steroid days

- Once your condition has been controlled, if you need steroids long term, your doctor will reduce the dose to the lowest possible level to reduce the risk of side effects.

Stopping steroids

When steroids are taken as treatment, they suppress the body's production of its own steroids, especially those made by the adrenal glands. These are small

Steroid production in the adrenal glands

When steroids are taken as treatment, they suppress the body's production of its own steroids, especially those made by the adrenal glands.

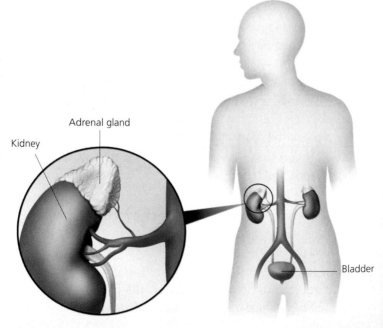

Kidney

Adrenal gland

Bladder

glands that sit on top of the kidneys and which produce steroids that control vital functions such as salt and water balance and blood pressure. If you stop taking steroids suddenly, you can become very ill because your adrenal glands need time to begin making their own steroids again. Therefore, steroids taken as treatment should always be tapered off gradually, to give the adrenal glands time to adjust.

Local steroid injections

If you have only one or two inflamed joints then steroids injected directly into the joints may be the best treatment. Many people with rheumatoid arthritis have repeated injections into their joints with great benefit. If the knee or the ankle is injected, it is safe to walk but you should rest the joint as much as possible for a day or two after the injection.

Steroid injections can also be given into painful and inflamed soft-tissue areas. This is a widely used and very effective form of treatment. Tennis elbow, tenosynovitis, and carpal tunnel syndrome are often completely relieved by the injection of a small amount of steroid.

The injected steroid remains at the site of the injection and is slowly dispersed. Very little is absorbed into the rest of the body and so, in contrast to steroids taken by mouth, local steroid injections produce very few side effects. Occasionally, some people experience an increase in their pain for 24 hours but this settles as soon as the steroid takes effect.

Local steroid injections carry a slight risk of wasting of the tissue and thinning of the skin at the injection site. This is seen as a small depression in the skin associated with loss of skin color, which is more obvious in people

A local injection of steroid

If you have only one or two inflamed joints then steroids injected directly into the joints may be the best answer. Here, the right shoulder is being injected from the back.

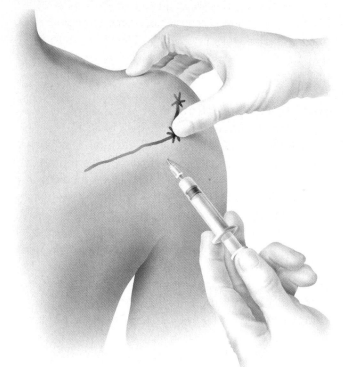

with pigmented skin. The only disadvantage of this is cosmetic but it is important to some people so they should always be aware of the risk.

Disease-modifying anti-rheumatoid drugs (DMARDs)

These are sulphasalazine, methotrexate, azathioprine, leflunomide (Arava), gold salts, penicillamine, and hydroxychloroquine, as well as the newer drugs etanercept (Enbrel), infliximab (Remicade) and adalimumab (Humira).

They form a very important group of drugs but are only used to treat widespread inflammatory arthritis, such as rheumatoid arthritis.

They are not used in other forms of arthritis and musculoskeletal conditions so information about them is included in the chapter on rheumatoid arthritis (see pages 21–9) rather than here.

Antidepressant drugs

Some people with chronic, painful conditions may develop depression, making the pain even harder to cope with. There are several antidepressant drugs that help to lift the mood and ease the pain. Interestingly, certain types of pain, such as neuralgia, are eased by antidepressants even in people who are not depressed.

These very useful drugs are not addictive and, although some of the older drugs may cause drowsiness, the newer ones do not.

Physiotherapy

Many people with joint problems are referred to a physiotherapist for treatment. Physiotherapists may be based in hospitals, some health centers, and in private clinics. Some are based in home care organizations in the community and can visit disabled people in their own homes. They are experts at maintaining the function of the musculoskeletal system—that is, they will help you maintain strength and movement and reduce pain.

After a course of treatment, the physiotherapist may give you an exercise program to work on at home, to continue the benefit of your treatment. But physiotherapy cannot work miracles. It is important for you to keep your part of the bargain. Lose weight if you are overweight, perform your exercises regularly, and take care of your joints.

Hydrotherapy

Hydrotherapy is physiotherapy performed in a warm swimming pool. It is very effective at relieving the discomfort of stiff, painful joints. The water supports the weight of your body and the warmth helps your muscles relax and your joints to move. A course of hydrotherapy can give prolonged benefit in conditions such as osteoarthritis of the hip and ankylosing spondylitis.

Surgery

Many people with arthritis assume all that a surgeon can do to help them is to replace a damaged joint. This is probably the most common operation, but it is by no means the only form of surgical treatment available. Your doctor may discuss the possibility of surgery with you if one or more joints have become so damaged, painful, and stiff that you can no longer use them effectively, despite taking painkillers and regular exercise.

Surgical options
Arthroscopy

This is a form of "keyhole" surgery usually performed under general anesthetic, but as an "ambulatory" procedure (that is, the patient is discharged from the hospital after the procedure, on the same day). It is used to diagnose and treat problems within a joint, most often injury to the knee. A thin tube passed

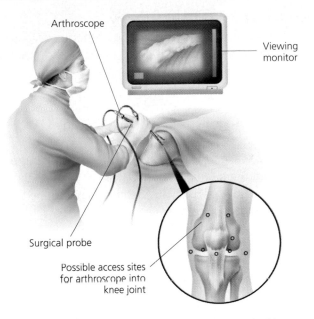

Arthroscope

Viewing monitor

Surgical probe

Possible access sites for arthroscope into knee joint

In arthroscopy, the inside of the joint is inspected with an arthroscope. Here the surgeon is operating on the knee joint.

through a small incision in the skin allows the surgeon to see into the joint. Other surgical instruments inserted through further small incisions allow the surgeon to perform small operations.

Synovectomy

This operation removes inflamed synovium from within joints and around tendons in people with rheumatoid arthritis. Although it can help to relieve symptoms and may slow the progress of the disease, it is not a cure, and the inflamed tissue often re-forms, sometimes quite quickly. For this reason, it is always used together with drug treatment.

Tendon and ligament surgery

Surgery can be performed to realign tendons or loosen tight tendon sheaths and even, in some cases, to repair broken tendons.

Osteotomy

If one area of a joint surface is badly damaged but other parts are still in a relatively good condition, surgery to realign the bone may redirect the pressure away from the damaged area. Osteotomy is sometimes used in younger people with arthritis to postpone the need for joint replacement.

Arthrodesis

This is surgery to fuse a joint so that it can no longer move. It abolishes pain but the joint is left completely

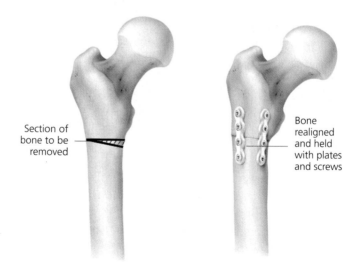

Section of bone to be removed

Bone realigned and held with plates and screws

An osteotomy creates a surgical fracture – in this case so that the hip may be realigned when the bone is rejoined.

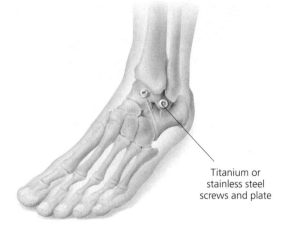

Titanium or
stainless steel
screws and plate

Arthrodesis means fusion of a joint to eliminate joint pain. Here the heel bone has been joined to a bone in the center of the foot using a metal plate.

stiff. It is a very useful operation for severe arthritis affecting the feet, ankles, wrists, and occasionally the spine.

Arthroplasty or joint replacement
Artificial joints for hips and knees have been widely used for over 20 years and have a very high success rate. In certain cases, shoulders, elbows, and finger joints can be replaced, although the surgery is technically more difficult.

Hip replacement
The two parts of a hip replacement are the metal femoral component (artificial upper thigh bone) and the plastic acetabular component (artificial hip socket). The combination of metal and plastic is very resistant to wear.

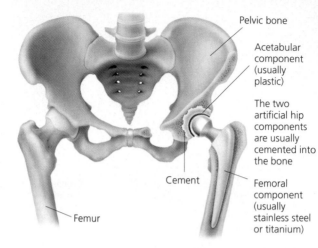

Pelvic bone

Acetabular component (usually plastic)

The two artificial hip components are usually cemented into the bone

Cement

Femoral component (usually stainless steel or titanium)

Femur

Knee replacement

The two parts of a knee replacement are the femoral component and the tibial component. Again, a combination of metal and plastic is used.

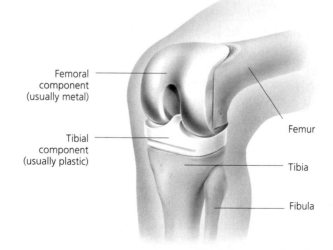

Femoral component (usually metal)

Tibial component (usually plastic)

Femur

Tibia

Fibula

Complementary medicine

Many people who have arthritis or rheumatism feel that they gain benefit from complementary medicines and use them as well as their conventional medication. This may be because orthodox treatment is unable to control their symptoms completely and also because they believe that complementary therapies are natural and safer.

Although there is some truth in this view, it is not the whole story, and there are other factors that you should bear in mind before deciding whether to try the complementary approach (see box on page 90).

In fact, it can be very difficult to make an objective assessment as to whether complementary methods and treatments are effective. Few have been scientifically tested, so there is little reliable evidence as to whether they actually work. The picture is complicated by the fact that the symptoms of arthritis may vary over time regardless of treatment, making it difficult to judge whether an improvement is the result of a particular treatment or simply part of the normal pattern of the disease.

Although many types of therapy are safe, you cannot always assume that this is so. In particular, you should be wary of herbal remedies imported from abroad and distributed by smallscale practitioners or stores. The quality of these products is not controlled and, in the past, some have been found to contain powerful drugs or even poisons such as heavy metals.

Copper bracelets

These are a traditional remedy for all kinds of aches and pains, but there is no real evidence that they are effective. However, they are unlikely to be harmful.

Using complementary medicines

- Do as much research as you can into the training and experience of the therapist. Reputable ones are likely to be registered with a regulatory body that monitors practitioners. Be especially wary of anyone who promises you a cure.

- Tell your doctor if you are using other types of treatment. Occasionally there may be undesirable interactions between conventional and complementary medicines.

- As with any medicine, always read the instructions on the package and do not exceed the recommended dose. It can be tempting to assume that "more is better," but this is unlikely to be the case.

- Never stop taking conventional treatments without consulting your doctor, especially if you are taking steroids, as stopping them suddenly can be dangerous.

- Try to relate the cost of treatment to its effectiveness—if you see no improvement after a reasonable time, there is no point in wasting your money. One way of doing this is to keep a diary of your symptoms for a month or so before starting any complementary treatment, and continue for another month once you are using it. You can then use this information to see whether you feel that the therapy is making any difference.

Glucosamine and chondroitin sulphate

These dietary supplements contain substances found naturally in the body which play a role in strengthening cartilage and help it to retain water. Some research has suggested that taking supplements may encourage damaged cartilage to repair itself, and even prevent cartilage damage in the first place, without causing side effects. Other research has shown no benefit. Some people find that the supplements help their pain but the ideal dose and formulation have not been identified, nor is it clear whether the effects will be long-lasting.

Fish oils
Fish oils and evening primrose oil contain essential fatty acids (called "essential" because the body cannot make them but must obtain them from food). There is now good scientific evidence that these oils can reduce inflammation in arthritis, although the effect is small. Cod liver oil contains essential fatty acids, together with vitamin D, which helps to absorb calcium. However, it also contains vitamin A and so should not be taken in large amounts as excess vitamin A can be dangerous.

Acupuncture
This traditional Chinese therapy involves inserting fine needles into the skin at certain carefully defined points to liberate the flow of "ki," sometimes called the "life force." Modern research suggests that it may help to reduce pain by stimulating the body to produce natural pain-killing chemicals called "endorphins." In China, acupuncture is used to treat a wide range of medical conditions and even to provide anesthesia for surgical operations.

In the west, there is some scientific evidence that it helps certain types of musculoskeletal pain and many physiotherapy departments now use it in a limited way. If you consult a private practitioner, make sure that he or she is registered. In skilled hands, the procedure is very safe.

Homoeopathy

Homoeopathy was devised as a system of medicine in the late nineteenth century and homoeopathic remedies are widely used today. The principle of treatment is that "like cures like." In other words, a homoeopath will choose remedies that, in larger amounts, would cause the symptoms being treated.

The actual choice of remedies will be based on your answers to extensive questioning about your history, symptoms, and personality. The remedies are made from substances extracted from plants, minerals, and animals, diluted many times over.

Homoeopaths hold that, as the substances are diluted, they become more "potent" and high-potency preparations are so diluted that they probably do not contain a single molecule of the original substance. Side effects and drug interactions are rare.

Osteopathy, chiropractic, and Alexander Technique

These are therapies with some similarities to physiotherapy, although they developed in very different ways. They are widely available privately but whether they are covered by your medical insurance will vary depending on your particular health policy and other factors. They can be particularly effective for spinal problems. Alexander Technique can be helpful in correcting faulty posture.

Practitioners teach how to use the body correctly and inhibit ingrained habits of poor posture and incorrect movement. Breathing techniques are also taught to aid movement.

Chiropractic is a variant of osteopathy. The two therapies are very similar and deal with biomechanical problems. They see pain and disability as arising from flaws in the function of the locomotor system. These flaws need not cause symptoms but may throw excessive strain on other parts of the locomotor system.

KEY POINTS

- Many different types of drug are useful in the treatment of locomotor problems

- Some people avoid drugs that could help them considerably because of misplaced fears—do not be afraid to take the drugs that your doctor recommends but, if you have concerns, talk to your doctor about them

- Complementary medicines and therapies can often help the symptoms of arthritis and rheumatism

- There is usually little scientific evidence that complementary medicines or therapies have a fundamental effect on diseases so, if they do not help your symptoms, they are best abandoned

- Always consult registered complementary practitioners and buy medicines from reputable shops and pharmacies

Living with arthritis and rheumatism

Exercise

Many people believe that they should rest their arthritic joints and that this will prevent further damage. In fact, the right kind of exercise is not only beneficial but essential for keeping the joints mobile and the muscles strong. Prolonged rest, on the other hand, usually leads to more stiffness and to weakness and wasting of the muscles, while having no effect on the pain.

Nevertheless, the wrong kind of exercise is worse than none at all. For example, touching your toes and "situps" put an enormous strain on the lumbar region of the spine.

You should also avoid "the squat"—bending your knees and hips from a standing position until your rear end touches your heels, then standing up again. This exercise really punishes your knees.

Do not rotate your head round like a windmill, hoping that this is a good exercise for your neck, because it can actually cause strain.

And lastly, never crack the joints in your fingers. What begins as a party trick can become a habit and can, over time, damage the joints.

Aim to include three types of exercise in your program:

- stretching exercises

- muscle-strengthening and exercises

- general fitness or aerobic exercises.

The program will also include a "weight-bearing" element to help strengthen your bones and reduce the risk of developing osteoporosis. A good exercise program should be part of your daily routine, whether or not you have arthritis.

Your exercise program

Always start with gentle exercises and then build up gradually. The right sort of exercise should not cause pain, so listen to your body and adjust your activities accordingly.

Stretching

Stretching involves putting each of your joints through a full range of movement every day. Begin at the top of your body and work downward so that no area is forgotten.

Neck

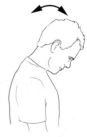

- Drop your head forward onto your chest and let it hang there for a few seconds.

- Then straighten up and drop your head to the side, again letting it hang for a few seconds. Repeat, dropping your head to the other side.

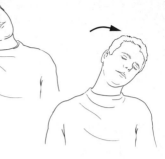

- Turn to look over your shoulder as far as you can and hold the position for a few seconds. Repeat, turning to the other side.

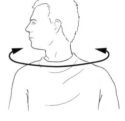

- Tip your head back as far as you can but do not force it, and this time do not hold the position for more than a second because you may feel dizzy.

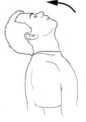

Shoulders

With your arms by your sides, rotate your shoulders in circles a few times, first forward and then backward.

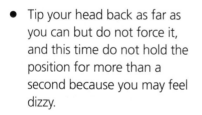

- Lift your arms up above your head, bringing them in against your ears and pushing them backward at the same time. Hold the position for a few seconds and then slowly bring them down sideways.

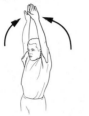
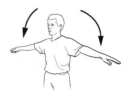

- Put your hands behind your back and clasp them. Then push your clasped hands backward, away from your trunk, and hold for a few seconds.

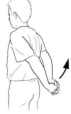

Elbows

- Straighten your elbows and then bend them up as far as they will go.

- Then, with your arms tucked into your sides and your elbows bent 90 degrees, turn your forearms so that your palms are facing upward and then downward.

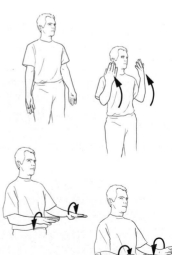

Wrists and hands

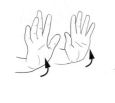

- Bend your wrists up and down as far as they will go.

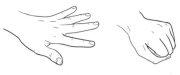

- Spread your fingers out hard and then clench your fists. Do this several times. If your fingers do not straighten fully, put your hand on a flat surface palm downward and very gently push the bent joints down with your other hand. Similarly, if your fingers do not close fully into a fist, very gently push them down with your other hand.

- Bring your thumb and index finger together in a pinch and then touch the tips of your other fingers in turn with your thumb. Repeat with your other hand.

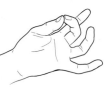

- The muscles in your hands can be strengthened by repeatedly squashing a soft rubber ball into your palm, allowing it to inflate fully between squashes.

Upper back (thoracic spine)

- Stand with your back against a wall and straighten your back so that the back of your head touches the wall. Hold for a few seconds.

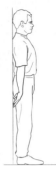

- Sit down and twist your trunk and shoulders to one side as far as you can, hold for a few seconds, and repeat to the other side.

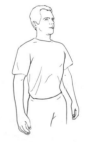

- Take a deep breath in, expanding your chest as much as possible, and hold for a few seconds.

Lower back (lumbar spine)

- Stand up straight and lean over to one side, running your hand down the side of your leg. Do not force the movement but just hang there for a few seconds. Repeat on the other side.

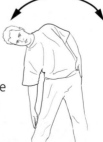

- Lie flat on the floor with your knees bent up. Lift your pelvis off the floor by tightening your stomach muscles, and hold for a few seconds.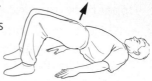

- Now straighten your legs out in front of you and push the small of your back against the floor, holding for a few seconds.

- Kneel on the floor on all fours. Make an arch of your back and then a hollow. Repeat several times (this exercise is known as "the cat").

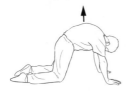

Hips

- Sit on the floor with your legs out in front of you, separate them out to the sides as far as they will go, and hold for a few seconds.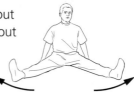

- Then bring your legs together and bend your knees up to your chest, one at a time if this is more comfortable. Hug your knees to your chest with your arms and hold them there for a few seconds (this is also a good exercise for your knees).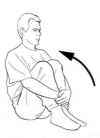

- Stand up and hold onto a chair back or table for support. Lift one leg and swing it back behind you as far as it will go. Repeat with the other leg.

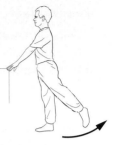

Knees

- Sit on a bed or on the floor with your back supported and your legs straight out in front of you. Push the backs of your knees hard against the surface, feeling the big quadriceps muscle in the front of your thigh tighten as you do so, and hold for a few seconds.

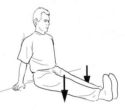

- Lift one leg up, keeping the knee straight, until your heel is about six inches above the surface. Once again, feel the quadriceps muscle working and hold for a few seconds. Repeat with the other leg.

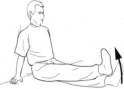

- Find a low step and step on and off, alternating with each leg.

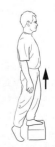

Ankles and feet

- Rotate your ankles in circles, first clockwise and then counter-clockwise.

- Bend your ankles up to bring your toes toward you and then bend them away from you, pointing your toes like a ballet dancer.

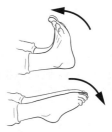

- Wiggle your toes.

Strengthening

Strengthening exercises work the muscles harder. Strong muscles are very important in helping to protect the joints from strain. Many of the exercises above will strengthen your muscles as well as stretching your joints.

More advanced muscle-strengthening exercises make the muscles work harder by lifting weights. The weights should be carefully chosen to suit you personally or the group of muscles being worked, so try to get advice from a qualified person such as a physiotherapist or trainer. Weights that cause pain are too heavy.

Aerobic

Aerobic exercise works your heart and lungs as well as some of your joints and increases your stamina. Activities such as swimming, brisk walking, and using an exercise bicycle are good examples. An exercise bicycle is particularly beneficial if you have arthritis in your hips or knees as the bicycle exercises these joints without them having to carry your weight at the same time. Swimming is a good choice if you are overweight because, again, the joints are exercised without having to support your body weight.

A moderate amount of exercise performed regularly, say two or three times a week, is much better for you than a blitz once a month, or only when you feel guilty. And even a small amount of exercise taken regularly, such as a daily 10-minute walk, is much better than doing nothing.

Protecting your joints

Besides regular exercise, looking after your joints also involves protecting them from unnecessary strain in your everyday activities. People with arthritis can avoid pain and preserve their independence by making changes in the way that they do things. This is not "giving in to arthritis" but simply good sense. Occupational therapists are experts in helping people to function as normally as possible, and advising on joint protection is one aspect of their work. They are based in hospitals and in community home healthcare organizations and, if necessary, they will visit you at home to advise on aids, appliances and adaptations. Aids for every aspect of daily living may be found in medical and surgical supply stores.

People with healthy joints can also benefit from simple advice on joint protection. Avoiding unnecessary strain makes good sense for them too. It can make difficult or tiring tasks easier and it can help to avoid problems in the future. An obvious place to start easing the strain is in the kitchen (see box below).

It is much easier on the hips and knees to get up from a high-seated chair with arms and out of a bath with handles. Shoes with soft, rubber cushioned soles act as shock absorbers and can protect the joints while walking. A cane can also be enormously helpful.

Walking with a cane

If you have problems with your knees or hips, a cane can make a huge difference to your comfort, confidence, and mobility. A cane, when used correctly, can take the load off an arthritic joint and help protect it from strain.

Tips in the kitchen

- A "bar" stool takes the weight off your legs when you are working at the sink, work surface, or ironing board.

- Steam irons are heavy and should be avoided if you have wrist, elbow, or shoulder problems.

- Saucepans with two handles share the load between both hands.

- Eye-level shelves and cabinets are less tiring than floor closets, as reaching up causes less strain than bending.

You can buy canes in pharmacies, medical supply stores, and other stores, and there are many different types. It is best to get expert advice about the right one from a physiotherapist or occupational therapist who can assess your needs and help you make the right choice.

Arthritis and the weather

At the first sign of cool, damp weather in the fall, many people with arthritis and rheumatism find that their symptoms get worse. On the other hand, during the summer months or when on vacation, their arthritis is much less troublesome. Sometimes it can seem as if the joints are acting as a barometer. Although this experience is very common, we do not know why joint pain and stiffness are so sensitive to changes in the weather. But we know that adverse weather conditions do not cause arthritis and they do not make existing arthritis worse.

Although people living in warm climates complain less of joint pain and stiffness, they develop the same forms of arthritis and often show abnormalities on their X-rays similar to those of people living in cool climates. Warmth is soothing and aids muscle relaxation and this is undoubtedly important in easing symptoms.

In warm weather and especially on vacation, people are often more active and the exercise is also beneficial to stiff, painful joints.

If you have arthritis, you should keep warm and try to maintain your levels of activity even when the weather is cold. A warm bath followed by a simple program of exercises can help enormously to reduce the pain and stiffness of arthritic joints.

Diet and arthritis

People often wonder if their diet has anything to do with their arthritis. The answer is, "probably not"! The one exception is gout (discussed on pages 30–5), where alcohol and foods containing large amounts of purines, such as liver, heart, kidney, and fish roe, can make the condition worse. Food allergies as a cause of arthritis are highly individual, difficult to test for, and probably very rare. However, if you feel that a certain food makes your symptoms worse, then you can perform an experiment called an "exclusion diet" to test this out (see box below).

There are lots of published "diets for arthritis," supported by glowing testimonials from people who claim that their particular diet "cured" their arthritis

Exclusion diet

- Keep a diary of your joint pain and stiffness for six weeks.
- For the first two weeks, eat a normal diet, including the suspect food.
- For the second two weeks, cut the suspect food out of your diet completely.
- For the third two weeks, include the suspect food in your diet again.
- If your symptoms improve during the middle two weeks when you exclude the food, and then get worse again when you reintroduce it during the last two weeks, then it is reasonable to conclude that the suspect food is making your symptoms worse.

and will cure yours too! Unfortunately, glowing testimonials do not amount to scientific evidence and you may waste a lot of money following a diet that has no good evidence to support it.

The best diet for arthritis is a healthy diet—one with a balance of protein, carbohydrates, and fats with plenty of fiber, vitamins, calcium, iron, and other minerals. A good diet will also help you to keep close to your ideal weight—and keeping your weight down is one of the best things that you can do to take the strain off your joints.

Arthritis and inheritance

Many people with arthritis want to know if the arthritis will "run in the family." It is certainly true that almost all forms have an inherited element—that is, if you have arthritis then your first-degree relatives (children and siblings) have an increased chance of developing it too. But for most forms of arthritis, the increased risk is still very small indeed. And even if they develop arthritis, it may still be mild, even if your arthritis is one of the severe forms. We cannot predict in advance who will and who won't develop arthritis and, more importantly, we cannot prevent it. The best advice is to lead a healthy life, take regular exercise, don't abuse your joints, and don't worry. Whatever form of arthritis you have, the chance that your child or grandchild will also have arthritis is very small.

Pain control

Pain should always be respected and constantly pushing yourself to continue activities that make it worse is counterproductive. On the other hand, too little activity is as bad as too much because it can leave

What should you weigh?

- The body mass index (BMI) is a useful measure of healthy weight
- Find out your height in inches (ins) and weight in pounds (lbs)
- Calculate your BMI like this

$$\text{BMI} = \left(\frac{\text{Your weight (lbs)}}{\text{Your height (ins)} \times \text{Your height (ins)}}\right) \times 703 \text{ (conversion factor)}$$

$$\text{e.g. } 23 = \left(\frac{160 \text{ lbs}}{70 \text{ ins} \times 70 \text{ ins}}\right) \times 703$$

- Males are recommended to try to maintain a BMI in the range 20.0 to 25.0
- Females are recommended to try to maintain a BMI in the range 18.7 to 23.8
- The chart below is an easier way of estimating your BMI. Read off your height and your weight. The point where the lines cross in the chart indicates your approximate BMI

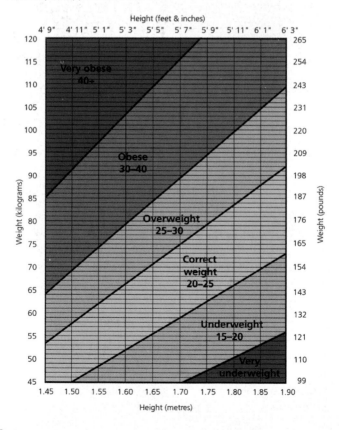

you with weakened muscles and encourage joints to stiffen and lose flexibility. There are many techniques for reducing pain besides drugs, and some of them you can easily try for yourself at home (see box, page 110).

The future

There are over 200 types of arthritis and, for many types, there is no single cause. Therefore, a single "cure for arthritis" is very unlikely to be found! But for people with arthritis of all kinds, a great deal of help is available and even people with severe arthritis can remain mobile and independent. In fact, most people with arthritis can lead normal lives.

On the other side of the coin, there is the fact that the population is living longer and people of all ages complain more about pain, stiffness, and other locomotor problems. What is the cause of this? Certainly, it does not seem that the more serious forms of arthritis, such as rheumatoid arthritis, are becoming commoner. Some of this increased stiffness, disability, and pain is undoubtedly caused by osteoarthritis, which is more common in older people. But much is also the result of body abuse—lack of exercise, overweight, poor posture, and overuse syndromes are the scourges of modern life in affluent societies. Abolishing these scourges would reduce not only locomotor problems but also diabetes, high blood pressure, and heart disease.

The remedy is largely in our own hands. You will notice how much we have emphasized the importance of exercise throughout this book. Exercise, exercise, and exercise are probably the three most important factors in keeping the joints healthy! Daily working lives are now much less active compared with 50 years ago. On

Practical pain control

Ice packs: you can buy cold packs to keep in the home freezer and use when you need them. If you use a bag of ice or a pack of frozen peas instead, wrap it in a dish towel or dry plastic bag to protect your skin, and apply it for no longer than 20 minutes. Cold packs are helpful for acute inflammation and swelling but avoid them if you have poor circulation or skin numbness.

Hot packs: these may be electric or ones you heat yourself (including microwaveable types) and are used in the same way as cold packs. Heat lamps work in a similar way, and don't neglect the traditional hot bath as a form of pain relief. Heat is good if you have deep aching pain, especially with muscle tension. Again, you shouldn't use hot packs if you have poor circulation or skin numbness because of the danger of accidental burns.

TENS (transcutaneous electrical nerve stimulation): this method of pain relief uses simple equipment to deliver a mild electric current through pads attached to the skin over painful areas. Stimulating nerves in this way blocks the pain sensations and prevents them reaching the brain. The equipment is safe and easy to use and is often especially helpful for hip, shoulder, and back pain. If you would like to try TENS then ask your physiotherapist.

Massage: if you have a partner, friend, or relative who is willing to learn how to give you a simple oil massage, this traditional form of therapy can be a big help in relieving pain, especially in the muscles. Either ask an expert to demonstrate or buy one of the many excellent books on the topic.

the other hand, exercise classes, swimming pools, and fitness facilities are now widely available, with activities to suit almost everyone, regardless of age. Find out about them today!

KEY POINTS

- The right sort of exercise, performed regularly, is essential for keeping your musculoskeletal system in the best possible condition

- The ideal is a balance of stretching for your joints, strengthening for your muscles, and aerobic exercise for stamina

Useful addresses

Where can I learn more?

We have included the following organizations because, on preliminary investigation, they may be of use to the reader. However, we do not have first-hand experience of each organization and so cannot guarantee the organization's integrity. The reader must therefore exercise his or her own discretion and judgment when making further inquiries.

Organizations with a commitment to providing useful patient information regarding Arthritis and Rheumatism:

Arthritis Foundation

1330 West Peachtree Street, Suite 100
Atlanta, GA 30309
Phone: 404-872-7100 or
800-568-4045 (WATS)
www.arthritis.org

National Institute of Arthritis and Musculoskeletal and Skin Diseases (NIAMS)

National Institutes of Health
1 AMS Circle
Bethesda, MD 20892–3675

Phone: 301-495-4484 or
877-22-NIAMS (226-4267) (WATS)
TTY: 301-565-2966
Fax: 301-718-6366
E-mail: NIAMSInfo@mail.nih.gov
www.niams.nih.gov

National Osteoporosis Foundation
1232 22nd Street N.W.
Washington, D.C. 20037–1292
Phone: 202-223-2226

**National Center for Complementary
and Alternative Medicine**
P.O. Box 7923
Gaithersburg, MD 20898
Phone: 301-519-3153 (international)
or 888-644-6226 (WATS)
TTY: 866-464-3615
Fax: 866-464-3616
E-mail: info@nccam.nih.gov
www.nccam.nih.gov

Scleroderma Foundation
300 Rosewood Drive, Suite 105
Danvers, MA 01923
Phone: 978-463-5843 or Toll-free: 800-722-HOPE (4673)
Fax: 978-463-5809

Spondylitis Association of America
P.O. Box 5872
Sherman Oaks, CA 91413
Phone: 818-981-1616 or 808-777-8199
E-mail: infor@spondylitis.org

NIH Osteoporosis and Related Bone Diseases-National Resource Center
1232 22nd St., NW
Washington, DC 20037–1292
Phone: 202-223-0344 or (800) 624-BONE
TTY: 202-466-4315
E-mail: NIAMSBoneInfo//www.osteo.org

National Fibromyalgia Association
2200 N. Glassell St., Suite A
Orange, CA 92865
Phone: 714-921-0150 Fax: 714-921-6920
www.fmaware.org

Lupus Foundation of America, Inc.
2000 L Street, N.W., Suite 710
Washington, DC 20036
Phone 202-349-1155
Fax 202-349-1156
www.lupus.org

Relevant Healthcare Professional Organizations:
American Medical Association
515 N. State Street
Chicago, Illinois 60610
Phone: 800-621-8335
http:www.ama-assn.org

American College of Rheumatology
1800 Century Place, Suite 250
Atlanta, GA 30345
Phone: 404-633-3777
www.rheumatology.org

American College of Physicians

190 N. Independence Mall

Philadelphia, PA 19106

www.acponline.org

American Academy of Family Physicians

P.O. Box 11210

Shawnee Mission, KS 66207–1210

Phone: 215-351-2400

www.aafp.org

American Academy of Orthopedic Surgeons

P.O. Box 2058

Des Plaines, IL 60017

Phone: 800-824-BONE (2663)

www.aaos.org

North American Spine Society (part of AAOS)

22 Calendar Court

2nd Floor

LaGrange, IL 60525

Phone: 877-SPINE-DR

E-mail: info@spine.org

www.spine.org

American Chiropractic Association

1701 Clarendon Boulevard

Arlington, VA 22209

Phone: 800-986-4636

www.amerchiro.org

American Osteopathic Association

142 East Ontario Street

Chicago, IL 60611

Toll-free phone: 800-621-1773
Phone: 312-202-8000
http://www.osteopathic.org/

**American Academy of Physical Medicine
and Rehabilitation**
330 North Wabash Ave., Suite 2500
Chicago, IL 60611–7617
info@aapmr.org

American Physical Therapy Association
1111 North Fairfax Street
Alexandria, VA 22314–1488
www.apta.org

American Occupational Therapy Association
4720 Montgomery Lane
P.O. Box 31220
Bethesda, MD 20824–1220
Phone: 301-652-2682
Fax: 301-652-7711
E-Mail: www.aota.org

The internet as a source of further information

After reading this book, you may feel that you would
like further information on the subject. The internet is,
of course, an excellent place to look and many websites
contain useful information about medical conditions,
related charities, and support groups.

It should always be remembered, however, that the
internet is unregulated and anyone is free to set up a
website and add information to it. Many websites offer
impartial advice and information that has been

compiled and checked by qualified medical professionals. Some, on the other hand, are run by commercial organizations with the purpose of promoting their own products. Others still are run by pressure groups, some of which will provide carefully assessed and accurate information whereas others may be suggesting medications or treatments that are not supported by the medical and scientific community.

Unless you know the address of the website you want to visit—for example,www.webmd.com—you may find the following guidelines useful when searching the internet for information.

Search engines and other searchable sites

Google (www.google.com) is the most popular search engine used in the United States, followed by Yahoo! (www.yahoo.com) and MSN (www.msn.com). Also popular are the search engines provided by Internet Service Providers such as AOL (www.aol.com).

In addition to the search engines that index the whole of the web, there are also medical sites with search facilities, which act almost like mini-search engines, covering only medical topics or even a particular area of medicine. Again, it is wise to look at who is responsible for compiling the information offered to ensure that it is impartial and medically accurate. One such site is the National Institute of Arthritis and Musculoskeletal and Skin Diseases Information Clearinghouse (www.niamis.nih.gov/hi/index.htm).

Search phrases

Be specific when entering a search phrase. Searching for information on "cancer" will return results for many

different types of cancer as well as on cancer in
general. You may even find sites offering astrological
information! More useful results will be returned by
using search phrases such as "lung cancer" and
"treatments for lung cancer." Both Google and Yahoo
offer an advanced search option that includes the
ability to search for the exact phrase; enclosing the
search phrase in quotes, that is, "treatments for lung
cancer," will have the same effect. Limiting a search to
an exact phrase reduces the number of results returned
but it is best to refine a search to an exact match only if
you are not getting useful results with a normal search.

Always remember the internet is international and
unregulated. It holds a wealth of valuable information
but individual sites may be biased, out-of-date, or just
plain wrong. Family Doctor Publications accepts no
responsibility for the content of links published in this
series.

Index

Your pages

We have included the following pages because they may help you manage your illness or condition and its treatment.

Before an appointment with a health professional, it can be useful to write down a short list of questions of things that you do not understand, so that you can make sure that you do not forget anything.

Some of the sections may not be relevant to your circumstances.

Health-care contact details

Name:

Job title:

Place of work:

Tel:

Name:

Job title:

Place of work:

Tel:

Name:

Job title:

Place of work:

Tel:

Name:

Job title:

Place of work:

Tel:

Significant past health events – illnesses/ operations/investigations/treatments

Event	Month	Year	Age (at time)

Appointments for health care

Name:

Place:

Date:

Time:

Tel:

Name:

Place:

Date:

Time:

Tel:

Name:

Place:

Date:

Time:

Tel:

Name:

Place:

Date:

Time:

Tel:

Appointments for health care

Name:

Place:

Date:

Time:

Tel:

Name:

Place:

Date:

Time:

Tel:

Name:

Place:

Date:

Time:

Tel:

Name:

Place:

Date:

Time:

Tel:

Current medication(s) prescribed by your doctor

Medicine name:

Purpose:

Frequency & dose:

Start date:

End date:

Medicine name:

Purpose:

Frequency & dose:

Start date:

End date:

Medicine name:

Purpose:

Frequency & dose:

Start date:

End date:

Medicine name:

Purpose:

Frequency & dose:

Start date:

End date:

Other medicines/supplements you are taking, not prescribed by your doctor

Medicine/treatment:

Purpose:

Frequency & dose:

Start date:

End date:

Medicine/treatment:

Purpose:

Frequency & dose:

Start date:

End date:

Medicine/treatment:

Purpose:

Frequency & dose:

Start date:

End date:

Medicine/treatment:

Purpose:

Frequency & dose:

Start date:

End date:

Questions to ask at appointments
(Note: do bear in mind that doctors work under great time
pressure, so long lists may not be helpful for either of you)

Questions to ask at appointments
(Note: do bear in mind that doctors work under great time pressure, so long lists may not be helpful for either of you)

Notes